Progesterone - Biological Function and Clinical Application

Edited by Zhengchao Wang

Published in London, United Kingdom

Progesterone - Biological Function and Clinical Application
http://dx.doi.org/10.5772/intechopen.110967
Edited by Zhengchao Wang

Contributors
Ali Shirinpur-Valadi, Crina Raluca Andrei, Florin Petrişor Posastiuc, Hisham Arab, Joaquim Esquerdo Ferreira, Lara Nogueira Silenciato, Marco Roberto Bourg de Mello, Mariana dos Santos Dutra Okada, Nicolae Tiberiu Constantin, Otávia Reis e Silva, Samuel Rodrigues Bonamichi do Couto, Seyedeh Khadijeh Abbasnia Zare, Shahram Sedaghathoor, Zhengchao Wang

First published in London, United Kingdom, 2024 by IntechOpen
IntechOpen is the global imprint of INTECHOPEN LIMITED, registered in England and Wales, registration number: 11086078, 167-169 Great Portland Street, London, W1W 5PF, United Kingdom

British Library Cataloguing-in-Publication Data
A catalogue record for this book is available from the British Library

Additional hard and PDF copies can be obtained from orders@intechopen.com

Progesterone - Biological Function and Clinical Application
Edited by Zhengchao Wang
p. cm.
Print ISBN 978-1-83769-416-7
Online ISBN 978-1-83769-415-0
eBook (PDF) ISBN 978-1-83769-417-4

For EU product safety concerns:
IN TECH d.o.o., Prolaz Marije Krucifikse Kozulić 3, 51000 Rijeka, Croatia,
info@intechopen.com or visit our website at intechopen.com.

Meet the editor

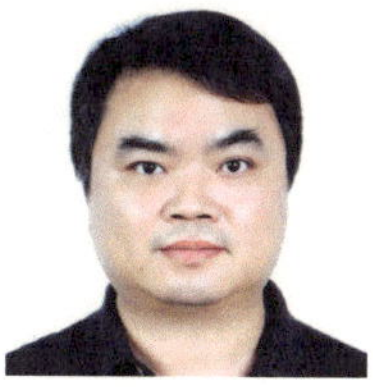

Dr. Zhengchao Wang is a full professor at the College of Life Sciences, Fujian Normal University, China. He is the Principal Investigator for the General Program for the National Natural Science Foundation of China and the Program for New Century Excellent Talents at the University of the Ministry of Education of China. He is also a team leader in the Fujian Provincial Key Laboratory for Developmental Biology and Neurosciences, Key Laboratory of Optoelectronic Science and Technology for Medicine of the Ministry of Education. He obtained his Ph.D. in 2008 and has many years of teaching and research experience. He has published more than 100 scientific papers and 10 books.

Contents

Preface

Progesterone is a natural steroid hormone secreted by the corpus luteum of the ovary. It not only regulates the female menstrual cycle but also has significant morphological effects on the estrogen-stimulated endometrium, which is necessary for maintaining pregnancy. Progesterone acts through progesterone receptors and is essential for mammalian embryo formation, development, and survival. In addition, progesterone induces the maturation and secretory activity of uterine endothelial cells, inhibits ovarian ovulation, and is linked to the pathogenesis of breast cancer.

In adult women, progesterone is low in concentration (< 2 ng/ml) during the menstrual cycle before ovulation. Levels increase to greater than 5 ng/ml during the luteal phase after ovulation. If pregnancy occurs, the progesterone concentration remains elevated during the early stages of pregnancy. When progesterone begins to be supplied by the placenta, the concentration increases to 100-200 ng/ml. The roles of progesterone include: (1) In the second half of the menstrual cycle, it promotes the growth of endometrial glands, uterine congestion, and endometrial thickening, preparing for fertilized egg implantation. It reduces the excitability of the pregnant uterus, inhibits its activity, relaxes smooth muscles, and enables safe embryo growth. (2) In conjunction with estrogen, it promotes the development of breast lobules and glands, enabling full breast development and preparing for lactation. (3) It closes the cervix, reduces mucus, thickens it, and makes it difficult for sperm to penetrate. At high doses, it inhibits ovulation by negatively affecting the hypothalamus and reducing pituitary gonadotropin secretion. (4) After ovulation, on the basis of hormone action, the endometrium continues to thicken and become congested, and the glands proliferate and branch, transitioning from a proliferative phase to a secretory phase, which is beneficial for the implantation of pregnant eggs and embryonic development. (5) It suppresses uterine contractions and reduces uterine sensitivity to oxytocin, ensuring safe fetal growth. (6) It competes against aldosterone to promote the excretion of Na and Cl and diuresis. (7) Progesterone has a mild warming effect, resulting in a higher basal body temperature in the luteal phase of the menstrual cycle compared to the follicular phase.

Progesterone also plays an important regulatory role during pregnancy and menopause. During pregnancy, the main function of progesterone is to suppress uterine contractions, maintain decidual response, and suppress immune response, ensuring fetal development and maintaining normal pregnancy. For menopausal women, progesterone supplementation can alleviate symptoms of hormone deficiency, delay aging, and, when combined with estrogen, provide better therapeutic effects. Long-term progesterone supplementation can prevent osteoporosis, protect brain function, and delay the onset of Alzheimer's disease. Progesterone also has new applications, including treating ureteral calculi, renal colic, chronic respiratory failure, male periodic psychosis, cirrhosis ascites, diabetes, sleep apnea syndrome, and menstrual asthma.

This book provides a comprehensive overview of the current state of the art in progesterone research to benefit women with related diseases. It aims to be meaningful to clinicians caring for women with progesterone disorders and researchers investigating these diseases. We thank all the authors for their contributions and hope this book supports clinicians and researchers involved in progesterone-related projects.

Dr. Zhengchao Wang
Provincial Key Laboratory for Developmental Biology and Neurosciences,
College of Life Sciences,
Fujian Normal University,
Fuzhou, China

Section 1

The Introduction of Progesterone

Chapter 1

Introductory Chapter: Progesterone

Zhengchao Wang

1. Introduction

Progesterone as a steroid participates in the female menstrual cycle of humans and other animals, supporting pregnancy and embryogenesis. It is one of the most essential progestogens. In non-pregnant women, progesterone is primarily secreted by corpus luteum (CL). During pregnancy, the placenta also secretes substantial amounts of progesterone. Additionally, the brain, liver, and adrenal glands secrete progesterone.

Steroid hormones are ancient molecules that regulate and interact with primitive cells, with cholesterol serving as a common precursor for all steroid hormones. The biosynthetic pathways of steroid hormones are consistent across various steroid-producing organs, such as the ovaries, testes, and placenta. However, the types and quantities of steroid hormones synthesized depend on specific enzymes in each organ.

Most gonadal-derived progesterone exerts its biological functions via blood transport, while most adrenal-derived progesterone is converted into glucocorticoids and androgens. The half-life of progesterone is very short, approximately 5 minutes, which is primarily metabolized in the liver and excreted in the urine.

Progesterone facilitates secretory endometrium transition, promotes blastocyst implantation, and is crucial for maintaining pregnancy. Progesterone is crucial to non-reproductive tissues, including mammary glands during pregnancy, and bones. Over the past decades, research has primarily focused on genomic/non-genomic mechanisms, enabling us to further understand its role and clinical applications in HR and diabetic neuropathy.

This chapter provides an overview of the biosynthesis, physiological functions, and regulatory mechanisms of progesterone, with the aim of enhancing the understanding of its safety and efficacy in various physiological and pathological contexts, thereby serving as an important reference for its clinical application.

2. The synthesis of progesterone

The synthesis of progesterone involves three consecutive steps [1–3]: (1) the STAR transports cholesterol to the inner mitochondrial membrane; (2) the P450SCC converts them into pregnenolone; (3) the 3β-HSD further converts them into progesterone. Notably, progesterone is the substrate of most steroids (**Figure 1**).

The STAR, P450SCC, and 3β-HSD are vital for the synthesis of progesterone [1–3]. Additionally, GST A1-1 and A3-3 synergistically produce progesterone with 3β-HSD. NR5A family members SF-1 and LRH-1 are also crucial [4, 5].

STAR acts as a cis-regulatory element for genes related to progesterone production, which is the steroidogenesis rate-limiting step [6]. Also, STAR regulation is

IntechOpen

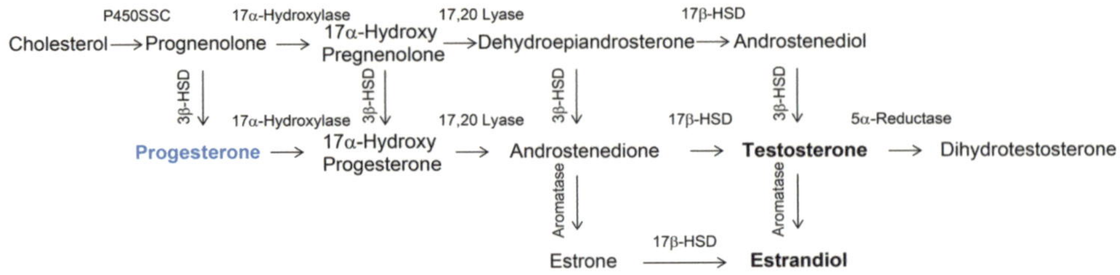

Figure 1.
The synthesis of progesterone and some other steroid hormones.

extensively characterized [7, 8]. NR5A can bind to the STAR promoter and then activate STAR transcription [7].

P450SCC is an enzyme crucial for the initial step in the steroidogenesis pathway, located within the mitochondria. Transgenic mice carrying a segment approximately 2.3 kb upstream of the human CYP11A1 gene exhibit tissue-specific and gonadotropin-dependent expression [9]. Alongside the NR5A binding site in the promoter, the construct also contains a cAMP response sequence and an adrenal enhancer as cis-regulatory elements within the 2.3 kb segment [10].

3β-HSD has two isoforms, placental HSD3B1 and gonadal HSD3B2 [11]. The promoter of human HSD3B2 contains the NR5A binding site, which is crucial to cAMP-stimulated transcription [11].

Besides above, several NR5A regulatory genes contribute to progesterone synthesis. Human GST, ALAS1, FDX1, and FDXR have been identified as proteins related to steroidogenesis.

3. The functions of progesterone

The role of progesterone can be categorized into two primary functions: its role in reproductive system tissues, such as the ovaries and endometrium, and its function in non-reproductive system tissues, including the central nervous system and bones (**Figure 2**).

3.1 The role of progesterone in reproductive system tissues

In the late 1960s, Ryan and Petro proposed the "two-cell two-gonadotropin theory" [12], which advanced the understanding of progesterone's role in the menstrual cycle. Specifically, LH stimulates follicular cells to synthetize androstenedione and subsequently converted into estrogen via follicle-stimulating hormone and the aromatase enzyme system [13]. Prior to ovulation, follicles synthesize estrogen and progesterone, which interact with membrane receptor PGRMC1 to promote follicle growth and inhibit apoptotic genes by directly affecting granulosa cells [14, 15]. Following the LH peak-induced ovulation, the CL forms [16]. During the follicular phase of the typical menstrual cycle, progesterone concentration remains below 1 ng/mL and then increases to 10 ~ 35 ng/mL within a few days after ovulation [17]. Additionally, PCOS ovarian luteinizing granulosa cells exhibit impaired ability to synthesize and secrete progesterone [18].

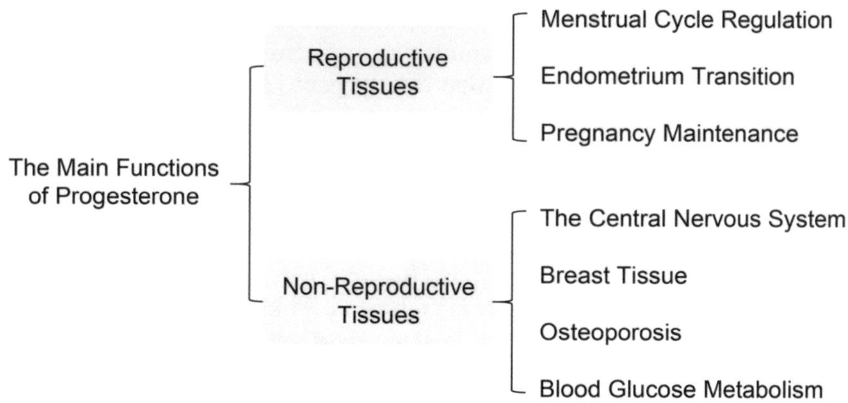

Figure 2.
The physiological and pathological functions of progesterone.

Progesterone is critical to the secretory endometrium transition. Throughout the menstrual cycle, the receptor expression of estrogen/progesterone in the endometrium varies. During the proliferative phase, PRs are primarily located in the epithelial cells of the endometrium. These receptors increase exponentially during ovulation in response to estradiol and subsequently decrease sharply [19, 20]. During the secretory stage, the endometrium undergoes combined effects of estrogen and progesterone. Progesterone halts endometrial growth by decreasing the cell mitotic activity [21, 22]. Additionally, progesterone exerts a protective effect on the endometrium of perimenopausal/postmenopausal women undergoing HRT [23].

During conception and early pregnancy, progesterone levels remain relatively stable but increase significantly in later stages, reaching 100–300 ng/mL. In the first nine-week pregnancy, progesterone is predominantly secreted by CL [23]. Subsequently, placental cells synthetize progesterone, making it the primary source after 12 weeks of gestation [24, 25]. Progesterone inhibits uterine contractions and suppresses immune responses at the maternal-fetal interface [25]. Approximately 35% of recurrent miscarriage cases are associated with luteal deficiency syndrome [24].

3.2 The role of progesterone in non reproductive system tissues

Progesterone significantly affects reproductive system tissues and also influences various other organs, thus being classified as a 'neurosteroid hormone' [26–28].

In CNS, progesterone regulates LH secretion within the hypothalamic-pituitary-adrenal axis, thereby developing a steroidogenesis feedback [29].

In breast tissue, progesterone facilitates the development of breast lobules and acini. Their mitotic activities are elevated in the follicular stage and decreased in the luteal stage. Progesterone also exerts a protective effect on breast tissue [30].

In blood glucose metabolism, progesterone can raise basal insulin and enhances its release following carbohydrate intake [31]. Progesterone secreted by the placenta elevates maternal blood glucose levels, which in turn increases fetal nutrient intake [28].

In osteoporosis, PRs express in osteoclasts and osteoblasts [32]. Progesterone inhibits bone resorption by directly stimulating calcitonin secretion and provides a nutritional benefit to bones similar to that of estrogens [32].

4. The mechanism of progesterone action

Progesterone primarily mediates its physiological and pathological effects by binding to specific progesterone receptors (PR) in the nucleus [30, 33]. PR is nuclear receptor, with two homologous receptors identified: 94 kDa PR-A and 114 kDa PR-B [30]. PR-A/B are transcripts encoded by a same gene, activated by distinct estrogen-induced promoters. Their functional characteristics and responses to progesterone differ [30]. For instance, PR-A can inhibit the transcriptional activity of other steroid hormone receptors, including estrogen receptors and PR-B [11, 33, 34]. Current research indicates that progesterone operates through two mechanisms: genomic/nuclear and non-genomic/extranuclear receptor pathways (**Figure 3**).

In the genomic receptor mechanism, PR-A/B share DNA and ligand-binding domains [34]. Lipophilic molecule progesterone diffuses through the membrane to interact with specific PRs in the nucleus, activating approximately 300 co-regulators influencing rRNA and protein synthesis [33]. The nuclear PRs require several minutes to hours to activate transcription, which serves as a primary regulator in reproductive function [34].

In non-genomic receptor mechanisms, progesterone rapidly activates multiple secondary messengers to exert its effects and is not affected by steroid nuclear receptor inhibitors [34]. The non-genomic receptor for progesterone located on the cell membrane is termed PGRMC1. Its interaction with SERBP1 mediates the anti-apoptosis of progesterone [35]. PGRMC1 and SERBP1 are implicated in ovarian cancer. Limited information is regarding PGRMC2, which is regulated by gonadotropins [35].

During progesterone action, these genomic/non-genomic mechanisms can collaborate to directly affect cells and tissues.

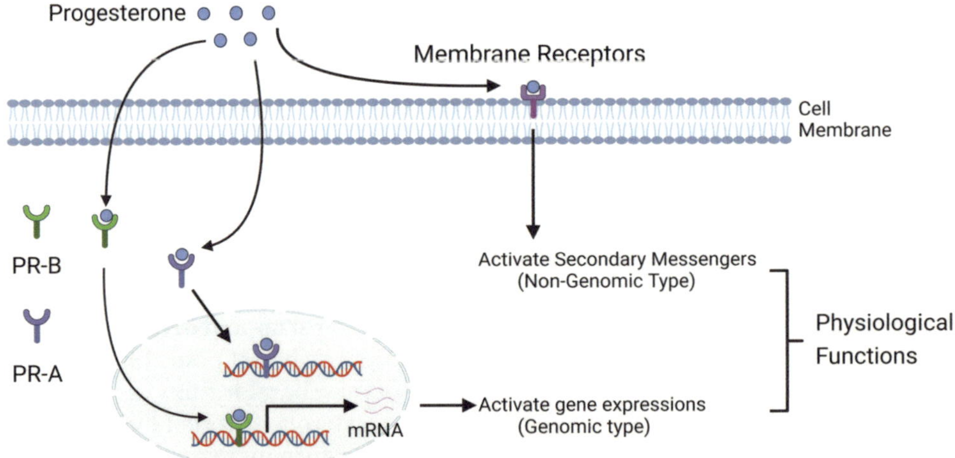

Figure 3.
The mechanism of progesterone action (created with BioRender.com).

5. Conclusion and prospect

Progesterone should be considered not only essential in the reproductive field but also a potential therapeutic agent for various clinical diseases, such as osteoporosis and diabetic neuropathy. Further understanding genomic/non-genomic receptor mechanisms will provide a comprehensive assessment of progesterone safety and efficacy in HRT, potentially reducing the risk of breast cancer. Additionally, a thorough understanding of progesterone's biological role will facilitate its safe and effective application across various scientific and medical fields.

Abbreviation

ALAS1	5-aminolevulinic acid synthase 1
3β-HSD	3β-hydroxysteroid dehydrogenase/Δ5-Δ4 isomerase
CNS	central nervous system
CL	corpus luteum
FDX1	ferritin 1
FDXR	ferritin reductase
GST	glutathione S-transferases
LH	luteinizing hormone
LRH-1	liver receptor homolog 1
NR5A	nuclear receptor 5A
P450SCC	cytochrome P450 cholesterol side-chain lyase
rRNA	ribosomal RNA
SERBP1	serpine mRNA binding protein I
PGRMC1	progesterone receptor membrane component-1
PR	progesterone receptor
SF-1	steroidogenic factor 1
STAR	steroidogenic acute regulatory protein

Author details

Zhengchao Wang
Provincial Key Laboratory for Developmental Biology and Neurosciences, College of Life Sciences, Fujian Normal University, Fuzhou, China

*Address all correspondence to: zcwang@fjnu.edu.cn

References

[1] Zhang Z, Shi C, Wang Z. The physiological functions and therapeutic potential of exosomes during the development and treatment of polycystic ovary syndrome. Frontiers in Physiology. 2023;**14**:1279469

[2] Zhang Z, Shi C, Wang Z. Therapeutic effects and molecular mechanism of chlorogenic acid on polycystic ovarian syndrome: Role of HIF-1alpha. Nutrients. 2023;**15**(13):2833

[3] Wang D, Tang Y, Wang Z. Role of sphingolipid metabolites in the homeostasis of steroid hormones and the maintenance of testicular functions. Frontiers in Endocrinology (Lausanne). 2023;**14**:1170023

[4] Zhang C et al. Liver receptor homolog-1 is essential for pregnancy. Nature Medicine. 2013;**19**(8):1061-1066

[5] Schimmer BP, White PC. Minireview: Steroidogenic factor 1: Its roles in differentiation, development, and disease. Molecular Endocrinology. 2010;**24**(7):1322-1337

[6] Stocco DM. StAR protein and the regulation of steroid hormone biosynthesis. Annual Review of Physiology. 2001;**63**:193-213

[7] Sugawara T et al. Steroidogenic factor 1-dependent promoter activity of the human steroidogenic acute regulatory protein (StAR) gene. Biochemistry. 1996;**35**(28):9052-9059

[8] Caron KM et al. Characterization of the promoter region of the mouse gene encoding the steroidogenic acute regulatory protein. Molecular Endocrinology. 1997;**11**(2):138-147

[9] Miller WL. Steroidogenic enzymes. Endocrine Development. 2008;**13**:1-18

[10] Shih MC et al. Regulation of steroid production: Analysis of Cyp11a1 promoter. Molecular and Cellular Endocrinology. 2011;**336**(1-2):80-84

[11] Simard J et al. Molecular biology of the 3beta-hydroxysteroid dehydrogenase/delta5-delta4 isomerase gene family. Endocrine Reviews. 2005;**26**(4):525-582

[12] Ryan KJ, Petro Z, Kaiser J. Steroid formation by isolated and recombined ovarian granulosa and tehcal cells. The Journal of Clinical Endocrinology and Metabolism. 1968;**28**(3):355-358

[13] Kobayashi M, Nakano R, Ooshima A. Immunohistochemical localization of pituitary gonadotrophins and gonadal steroids confirms the 'two-cell, two-gonadotrophin' hypothesis of steroidogenesis in the human ovary. The Journal of Endocrinology. 1990;**126**(3):483-488

[14] Peluso JJ. Progesterone receptor membrane component 1 and its role in ovarian follicle growth. Frontiers in Neuroscience. 2013;**7**:99

[15] Yuan XH et al. Progesterone maintains the status of granulosa cells and slows follicle development partly through PGRMC1. Journal of Cellular Physiology. 2018;**234**(1):709-720

[16] Frederick JL, Shimanuki T, diZerega GS. Initiation of angiogenesis by human follicular fluid. Science. 1984;**224**(4647):389-390

[17] Rangel PL et al. Testosterone stimulates progesterone production and STAR, P450 cholesterol side-chain cleavage and LH

receptor mRNAs expression in hen (Gallus domesticus) granulosa cells. Reproduction. 2009;**138**(6):961-969

[18] Yang J, Chen C. Hormonal changes in PCOS. The Journal of Endocrinology. 2024;**261**:1

[19] Gomes VCL et al. Estrogen and progesterone receptors are dysregulated at the BPH/5 mouse preeclamptic-like maternal-fetal interface. Biology (Basel). 2024;**13**(3):192

[20] Lessey BA et al. Immunohistochemical analysis of human uterine estrogen and progesterone receptors throughout the menstrual cycle. The Journal of Clinical Endocrinology and Metabolism. 1988;**67**(2):334-340

[21] Bildik G et al. Cholesterol uptake or trafficking, steroid biosynthesis, and gonadotropin responsiveness are defective in young poor responders. Fertility and Sterility. 2022;**117**(5):1069-1080

[22] Rantala MH et al. Endometrial expression of progesterone, estrogen, and oxytocin receptors and of 20alpha-hydroxysteroid dehydrogenase and cyclooxygenase II 2 and 5 days after ovulation in induced short and normal estrous cycles in dairy cows. Theriogenology. 2014;**81**(9):1181-1188

[23] Kissinger D. Hormone replacement therapy perspectives. Frontiers in Global Women's Health. 2024;**5**:1397123

[24] Cavoretto PI et al. Prospective longitudinal cohort study of uterine arteries Doppler in singleton pregnancies obtained by IVF/ICSI with oocyte donation or natural conception. Human Reproduction. 2020;**35**(11):2428-2438

[25] Schneider MA, Davies MC, Honour JW. The timing of placental competence in pregnancy after oocyte donation. Fertility and Sterility. 1993;**59**(5):1059-1064

[26] Maguire JL, Mennerick S. Neurosteroids: Mechanistic considerations and clinical prospects. Neuropsychopharmacology. 2024;**49**(1):73-82

[27] Goyette MJ et al. Sex hormones, neurosteroids, and glutamatergic neurotransmission: A review of the literature. Neuroendocrinology. 2023;**113**(9):905-914

[28] Taraborrelli S. Physiology, production and action of progesterone. Acta Obstetricia et Gynecologica Scandinavica. 2015;**94**(Suppl. 161):8-16

[29] Liang G et al. Menopause-associated depression: Impact of oxidative stress and neuroinflammation on the central nervous system-A review. Biomedicines. 2024;**12**(1):184

[30] Conneely OM, Mulac-Jericevic B, Arnett-Mansfield R. Progesterone signaling in mammary gland development. Ernst Schering Foundation Symposium Proceedings. 2007;**1**:45-54

[31] Shao J, Qiao L, Friedman JE. Prolactin, progesterone, and dexamethasone coordinately and adversely regulate glucokinase and cAMP/PDE cascades in MIN6 beta-cells. American Journal of Physiology. Endocrinology and Metabolism. 2004;**286**(2):E304-E310

[32] Toumba M et al. Estrogen receptor signaling and targets: Bones, breasts and brain (review). Molecular Medicine Reports. 2024;**30**(2):144

[33] Lonard DM, Lanz RB, O'Malley BW. Nuclear receptor coregulators and

human disease. Endocrine Reviews. 2007;**28**(5):575-587

[34] Gellersen B, Fernandes MS, Brosens JJ. Non-genomic progesterone actions in female reproduction. Human Reproduction Update. 2009;**15**(1):119-138

[35] Koensgen D et al. Expression analysis and RNA localization of PAI-RBP1 (SERBP1) in epithelial ovarian cancer: Association with tumor progression. Gynecologic Oncology. 2007;**107**(2):266-273

Section 2

The Biological Function of Progesterone

Chapter 2

Progesterone and Steroids In/On Plants

Shahram Sedaghathoor, Seyedeh Khadijeh Abbasnia Zare and Ali Shirinpur-Valadi

Abstract

Plants and animals contain many steroid compounds that act as signaling molecules during complicated growth and development processes. Mammal sex hormones (MSHs), such as progesterone, estrogen, and testosterone, are another class of steroids. These hormones play an important role in regulating the mammals' growth and reproduction processes as well as organic and inorganic metabolism. Steroid sex hormones, such as progesterone, beta-estradiol, and testosterone, support plant life processes including callus expansion, cytokinesis, root and shoot enlargement, and pollination in plants and have appropriate effects on handling abiotic stresses. An interesting impact of MSH is its capability in improving plant resistance to various abiotic stresses. MSH treatment extensively can reduce the adverse effects of environmental stress by promoting the activity of antioxidant enzymes, including superoxide dismutase (SOD), peroxidase (POX), and catalase (CAT), and improving proline production.

Keywords: mammal sex hormones (MSHs), brassinosteroid, environmental stress, phytoestrogens, androgen

1. Introduction

Mammalian sex hormones, including estrogens, androgens, and progesterone, are classified as steroids due to their tetracyclic triterpanes (sterane) structure. The diversity of steroids within animals and plants is dictated by the arrangement and kinds of functional groups linked to the sterane. In mammals, these steroid sex hormones play a crucial role in regulating development, reproduction, as well as mineral and protein metabolism [1]. The discovery of estrogen in plants dates back to 1926 when Dohrn et al. [2] first identified it. However, these early findings were considered preliminary due to the imperfect detection methods available at the time. Subsequent to these discoveries, a plethora of studies analyzing human and animal sex hormones in plants were published between the initial findings and the 1980s.

Certain analytical techniques, such as the Kober color reaction, have been subject to critical assessment. For instance, Van Rompuy and Zeevaart, in 1979, highlighted the need for more sensitive investigative methods for detecting estrogen-like substances in plants. The continuous evolution of detection methods has been crucial in advancing our understanding of the presence and role of sex hormones in plant biology [1]. Extensive research on the presence of mammalian steroids in plants (128 species from over 50 families) was conducted through radioimmunoassay in 1989 [3]. Steroids such as androsterone, progesterone, testosterone, dihydrotestosterone, estrone, and 17β-estradiol have been found in a significant number of plant species. In fact, over 80% of the studied species contained androsterone and progesterone, while 70% contained androgens, and 50% contained estrogens. The levels of steroids can vary significantly throughout plant growth and are influenced by species, cultivar, and plant organ [1]. During the latter part of the twentieth century, scientists worldwide actively sought to confirm the existence of animal steroid hormones in plants. Indeed, all animal steroid hormones or their analogs were discovered in plants. Moreover, the external application of animal hormones was shown to influence growth, development, and sexual characteristics in plants [4, 5]. These findings regarding the growth-regulating impact of animal steroid hormones in plants spurred the exploration of naturally occurring steroidal compounds that regulate growth. These investigations ultimately led to the identification of brassinosteroids, the sixth category of plant hormones found universally in plants.

2. Brassinosteroids: a novel phytohormone

Brassinosteroids (BRs) are a class of growth-promoting steroidal phytohormones. BRs are a distinct group of plant polyhydroxysteroids that bear a striking resemblance to cholesterol-derived animal steroid hormones. These compounds are found throughout the plant kingdom and have the ability to induce significant physiological changes in various plant species when applied externally. Surprisingly, despite their discovery in rapeseed pollen, BRs did not gain recognition as crucial plant hormones for more than 25 years. The delayed acknowledgment of the importance of BRs highlights the complexity of plant hormone research and the intricacies of understanding plant physiology. As scientists continue to delve deeper into the role of BRs in plant growth and development, it becomes increasingly clear that these compounds play a significant role in regulating various physiological processes [6].

Brassinosteroids (BRs), a class of steroid plant hormones, play a crucial role in regulating various developmental processes in plants, such as root and shoot growth, vascular differentiation, fertility, flowering, seed germination, and response to environmental stresses. Over the past 40 years, research has extensively delved into the BR biosynthetic pathways using forward- and reverse genetics approaches. These pathways have shed light on the structure of free BRs, which typically consist of 27, 28, or 29 carbons. These carbon structures bear resemblance to sterols, as they share common alkyl substituents. BRs are derived from sterols with similar side chains. The structural differences among various BRs, specifically C27-BRs, C28-BRs, and C29-BRs, are indicative of their distinct origins from different sterols such as cholesterol, campesterol, 24-epicampesterol, 24-ethylenecholesterol, and sitosterol. Furthermore, variations in substituents at specific carbon positions further differentiate BRs derived from these sterols. For instance, the classification of C27-BRs without a substituent at C-24 as derivatives of cholesterol, and C28-BRs with specific substituents as originating from campesterol, 24-epicampesterol, or 24-ethylenecholesterol, along with C29-BRs with an α-ethyl group being derived from sitosterol, underscores the intricate biochemical pathways involved in the synthesis of sterols, whereas those with a methylene group at C-24 and an additional methyl group at C-25 are derived from 24-methylene-25-methylcholesterol. Commonly, brassinosteroids are synthesized through pathways dependent on cycloartenol and cycloartanol. Notably, more than 17 compounds have been identified as inhibitors of BR biosynthesis, with specific target reactions within the pathway elucidated for nine inhibitors like brassinazole and YCZ-18 [7].

Brassinosteroids (BRs) have been identified as the 6th group of phytohormones, with approximately 70 naturally occurring compounds belonging to this group. These compounds, including brassinolide (BL), are structurally similar to androgens, estrogens, corticoids, and ecdysteroids. BRs are found in both lower and higher plants, particularly in angiosperms, and are present in various plant organs. These hormones are essential for the development and growth of plants, as they trigger various morphological and physiological responses. Among these hormones, brassinosteroids (BRs) play a crucial role in enhancing plant tolerance against abiotic and biotic stressors. BRs help plants adapt to adverse environmental conditions, allowing them to thrive and survive in challenging situations. Their importance in plant biology cannot be overstated, as they contribute significantly to the overall health and resilience of plants. In conclusion, understanding the role of hormones such as BRs is vital for improving crop productivity and sustainability in agriculture [7–9].

2.1 BRs biosynthesis

BRs, a group of phytohormones, are categorized as C27, C28, or C29 steroids based on their C-24 alkyl substituents. Among them, brassinolide, a C28 brassinosteroid, has been found to possess the most potent biological activity [10]. The discovery of two distinct biosynthesis pathways (the early and late C-6 oxidation pathways) for brassinolide in cultured *Catharanthus roseus* cells has provided valuable insights into the production of this important plant hormone and the complex mechanisms governing plant growth and development [11, 12]. The validation of each step within these pathways was achieved through the conversion of labeled brassinosteroids. Research indicates the occurrence of cross-talk between these parallel pathways, underscoring the complexity of brassinosteroid biosynthesis. Additionally, an early C-22 oxidation pathway has been identified to occur at the initial stages of biosynthesis. These intricate biosynthetic pathways form a network that appears to be prevalent across the plant kingdom, with similar pathways observed in a diverse range of plants, including *Arabidopsis*, rice, pea, and zinnia [11]. In tomato and tobacco plants, the late C-6 oxidation pathway is the primary route for the synthesis of brassinosteroids (BRs). This is due to the fact that the endogenous BRs found in these species consist solely of members from the late C-6 oxidation pathway. Unlike other plants where both early and late pathways are involved in BR synthesis, tomato and tobacco plants rely exclusively on the late C-6 oxidation pathway. This unique characteristic sets them apart from other plant species and highlights the importance of understanding the specific pathways involved in BR synthesis in different plants. Further research into the regulation and significance of the late C-6 oxidation pathway in tomato and tobacco plants could provide valuable insights into their growth and development processes [11].

The biosynthesis of brassinosteroids (BRs) involves three distinct pathways that result in the production of C27-, C28-, or C29-type BRs (**Figure 1**). The initial steps of synthesis are shared among these pathways and can occur through either the

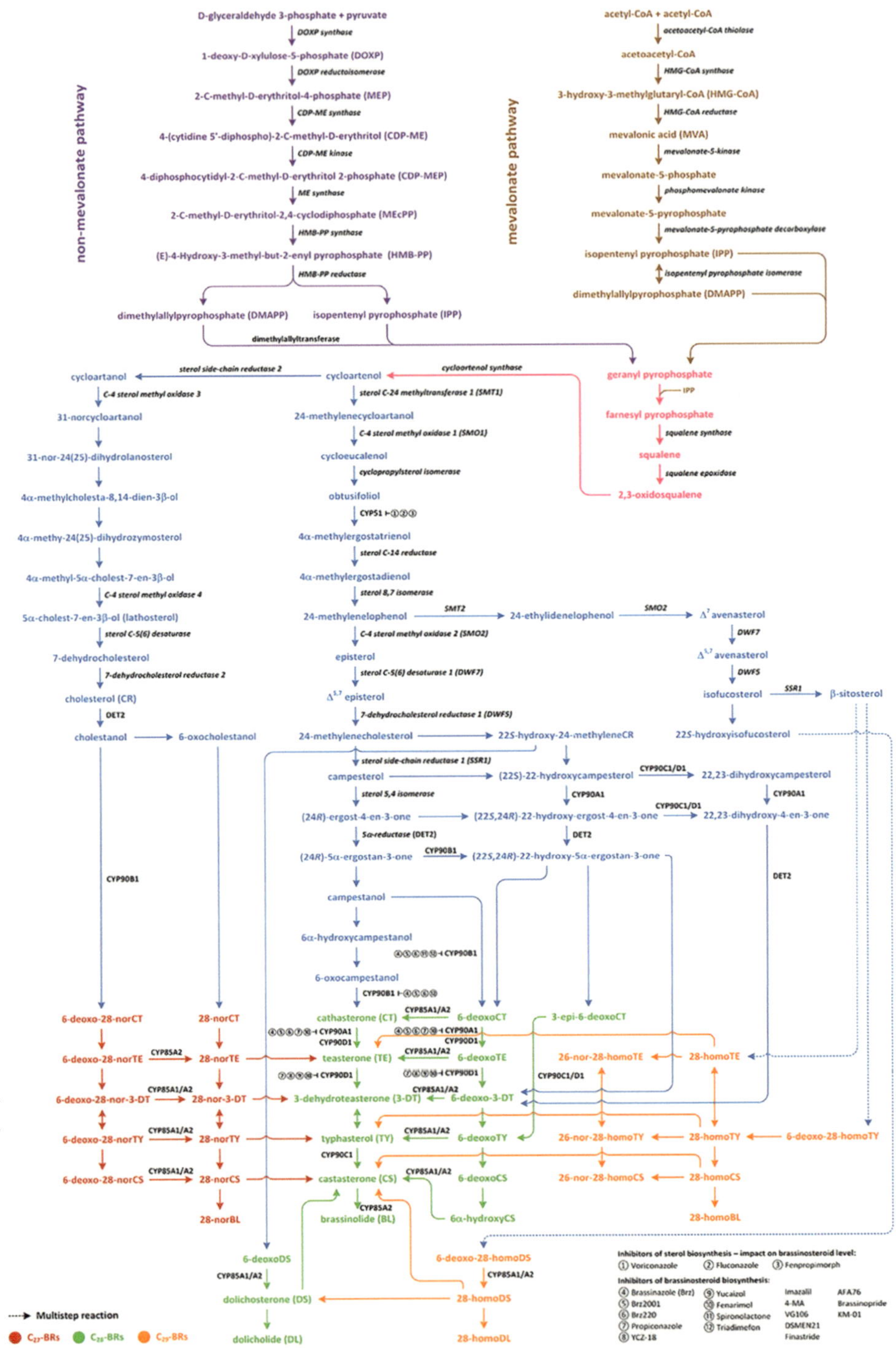

Figure 1.
Brassinosteroids biosynthesis and their sterol biosynthetic precursors [7].

mevalonate (MVA) or non-MVA pathway. However, the later stages of biosynthesis, which are cycloartenol- and cycloartanol-dependent, differentiate the BR biosynthesis pathways. The C28-BR biosynthesis pathway, primarily studied in *Arabidopsis thaliana*, has provided significant insights into the reactions, enzymes, and genes involved in BR production. This pathway involves the synthesis of campesterol and 22a-hydroxycampesterol. C27-BRs are derived from cholesterol (CR) and culminate in the production of 28-norBL, while C29-BRs originate from b-sitosterol and result in 28-homoBL. Despite the progress made in identifying compounds along these pathways, not all indirect compounds have been fully characterized yet (**Figure 1**) [7].

In the realm of plant biology, the oxidation/hydroxylation steps in the BR biosynthetic pathway play a crucial role, being catalyzed by cytochrome P450 enzymes. Traditionally, it was thought that brassinolide is synthesized from campesterol through campestanol (CN) in the initial BR biosynthetic pathway [13]. P450s catalyze the stereospecific oxidation of unactivated hydrocarbons. They are found in over 5000 species. In plants, *Arabidopsis thaliana* has 245 P450 genes, *Oryza sativa* has 334, *Vitis vinifera* has 316, *Glycine max* has 332, *Physcomitrella patens* has 71, *Chlamydomonas* has 40, and *Volvox* has 19. The number of plant P450s surpasses that of *Drosophila* (87 genes) and humans (56 genes). P450 is a hemoprotein featuring heme iron at its active center, along with a cysteine-derived thiolate anion coordinated with the heme iron. The maximum absorption band (Soret band) of reduced P450 is approximately 420 nm. Upon carbon monoxide binding to the heme iron Fe (II) in reduced P450, the Soret band shifts to 450 and 380 nm (the origin of the name "pigment 450 nm"). Plant P450s are located in the endoplasmic reticulum membrane and facilitate substrate oxidation by activating molecular oxygen with NADPH-P450 reductase. Notably, P450 serves as a common target for fungicides and plant growth substances [13–15].

2.2 BRs biosynthesis inhibitors

The discovery of brassinazole as a potential BR-biosynthesis inhibitor marked a significant advancement in the field of plant research. Through investigations on small molecules that induce BR-deficiency-like phenotypes in *Arabidopsis*, researchers were able to pinpoint brassinazole as the primary candidate for inhibiting BR biosynthesis. Studies have shown that treatment with brassinazole effectively reduces BR content in plant cells by binding directly to the DWF4 protein, a cytochrome P450 monooxygenase responsible for catalyzing 22-hydroxylation of the side chain of BRs. The findings strongly indicate that brassinazole acts as a potent inhibitor of the natural synthesis of BRs, with effects resembling conditional mutations in BR biosynthesis. The identification of brassinazole and other known inhibitors represents a crucial step forward in understanding the intricate mechanisms governing plant growth and development [11, 16, 17].

Today, seventeen inhibitors (KM-01, brassinozole (Brz), Brz2001, Brz220, propiconazole, YCZ-18, yucaizol, fenarimol, spironolactone, triadimefon, imazalil, 4-MA, VG106, DSMEM21, finastride, AFA76, and brassinopride) have been known (**Figure 2**); however, the activity position of just 9 inhibitors is recognized [7].

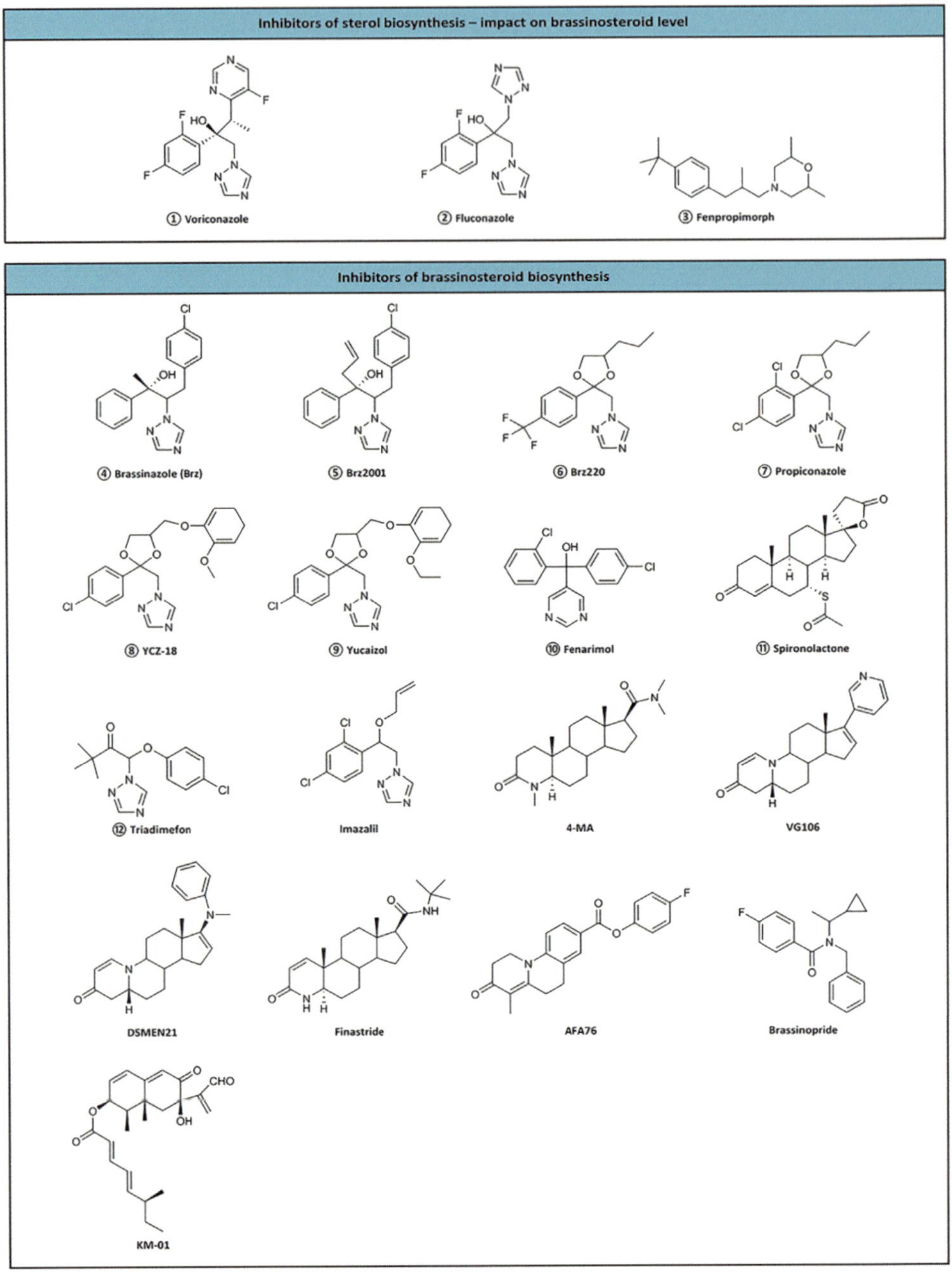

Figure 2.
Inhibitors of biosynthesis of sterol and BR. Numbered compounds have a recognized activity site [7].

The following are the action sites of inhibitors:

- campestanol—6-deoxoCT for brassinazole, Brz2001, Brz220, triadimefon, and spironolactone;
- 6-deoxoCT—6-deoxoTE for brassinazole, Brz2001, Brz220, propiconazole, and fenarimol;

- 6-deoxoTE—6-deoxo-3DT for YCZ-18, yucaizol, propiconazole, and fenarimol;
- 6-oxocampestanol—CT for brassinazole, Brz2001, Brz220, and triadimefon;
- CT—TE for brassinazole, Brz2001, Brz220, propiconazole, and fenarimol;
- TE—3DT for YCZ-18, yucaizol, propiconazole, and fenarimol (**Figure 1**) [7, 18].

The first stated BR inhibitor, i.e., KM-01, was sequestered from a microbiological media. KM-01 disabled BR activity in a rice lamina. Regardless of the uncertain location of activity, KM-01 displays extremely strong activity. But, brassinazole (Brz) represents the primary particular BR synthesis inhibitor, which inhibits the exchange of campestanol to 6-deoxoCT, 6-deoxoCT to 6-deoxoTE, 6- oxocampestanol to CT, and CT to TE in the BR biosynthetic same reactions [7, 16–18]. Brz and Brz2001 can induce morphological changes, including dwarfism, altered leaf color, and curling in de-etiolated barley. Brz reduced the amount of BRs in the shoots of barley, but not in roots. The inhibitory impact of Brz on plant growth is retreated by exogenous BR. Propiconazole, a triazole compound, also affects similar to Brz. New triazole-type BR biosynthesis inhibitors, YCZ-18 and yucaizol, bind to the CYP90D1 enzyme and prevent the BR-induced cell growth. On the other hand, just BL denies the inhibition influence of YCZ-18 or yucaizol [7, 11, 18].

3. Estrogens and androgens in plants

Steroid hormones in mammals are categorized into five classes according to their construction and natural functions (**Figure 3**). These groups include androgens, estrogens, which are male and female sex hormones, mineralocorticoids and glucocorticoids, necessary for regulating the body's homeostasis, and progestins, with progesterone playing

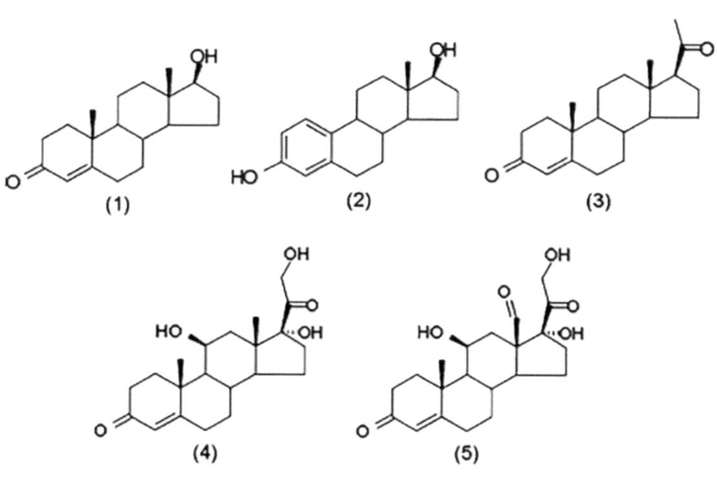

Figure 3.
Constructions of steroids which are main groups of mammalian steroid hormones: 1, testosterone (androgens), 2, estradiol (estrogens), 3, progesterone (progestins), 4, cortisol (glucocorticoids), 5, aldosterone (mineralocorticoids) [19].

a crucial role in the onset and maintenance of pregnancy [19]. Estrogen is a group of sex hormones that play a role in developing and controlling the female reproductive system and secondary sexual traits. Three main natural estrogens with hormonal effects are estrone (E1), estradiol (E2), and estriol (E3). Estetrol (E4), another estrogen, is only produced during pregnancy. An androgen is a natural or synthetic steroid hormone that controls the development and upkeep of male traits in vertebrates by binding to androgen receptors. The primary androgen in males is testosterone. Dihydrotestosterone (DHT) and androstenedione are equally significant in male development.

The presence of endogenous estrogens and androgens may be questioned due to their small amounts in plants. Additionally, various metabolites in the plant extract can impede analysis and result in inaccurate outcomes. According to this subject, in more progressive analytical procedures, emphasis should be placed on appropriately cleaning the sample. These compounds (androgens and estrogens) are found in plants at the pg. and ng levels [20].

Khaleel et al. [21] found that 17β-estradiol varied in concentration, from 14 pg/g F.W. $\times 10^{-1}$ in a bisexual tree (branch 1, November) to 2624 pg/g F.W. $\times 10^{-1}$ in the generative buds of a bisexual tree *Populus tremuloides* (March). They observed that in catkins, hormone concentrations were higher before anthesis, peaked during flowering, and then decreased as the flowers matured. These increases were associated with sporogenesis and gametophyte development. Seasonal variation in 17β-estradiol concentration was noted, along with the effect of radiation circumstances and the specific plant tissue being investigated. Dormant winter parts had minor 17β-estradiol than spring active organs, and twigs developing in more strong radiation contained further 17β-estradiol content. Fluctuations in 17β-estradiol and testosterone were also found in *Actinidia* pollen by researchers [22].

Hormone levels rose during pollen germination, specifically during tube organization, emergence, and elongation phases. The process of pollen germination in kiwifruit involves fluctuations in hormone levels, particularly 17β-estradiol and testosterone, during key phases such as tube organization, emergence, and elongation. The presence of 17β-estradiol in kiwifruit pollen can rise from nearly undetectable levels in ingeminated pollen to around 4 ng/mg pollen after 90 minutes of germination, while testosterone levels can vary from 0 to 2.5 ng/mg pollen. Furthermore, the introduction of bisphenol A has been shown to elevate the levels of both 17β-estradiol and testosterone. Excessive concentrations of exogenous 17β-estradiol and testosterone have been found to hinder kiwifruit pollen germination, suggesting that environmental contamination by bisphenol A could potentially disrupt plant fertility by affecting steroid content. Some studies have indicated that the presence of estrogens and androgens in plants may pose risks to both humans and animals [20–23]. For instance, research by Lu et al. [24] revealed varying levels of 17β-estradiol in vegetables and fruits, with concentrations ranging from 1.3 to 2.2 ng/g F.W. across different species, while estrone was detected in smaller amounts. Notably, the intake of 17β-estradiol in children from plant-based foods could exceed recommended daily limits, highlighting the importance of monitoring hormone levels in food sources as discussed by Palacios et al. [25].

Zeitoun and Alsoqeer [23] studied the sex steroid hormones in alfalfa and their following impacts on camel reproduction. Testosterone was recognized in *Cakile arabica* (3.69 ng/g D.W.) and Dwarf papyrus sedge (2.97 ng/g D.W.) but not in Greater plantain, Arfaj, Buffel grass, and Alfalfa. Additionally, 17β-estradiol was reported in prickly lettuce (379 pg/g D.W.), Rocket (247 pg/g D.W.), and *Heliotropium bacciferum* (229 pg/g D.W.) but not in Broom bush, Arfaj, and plumose needlegrass. Based on the results, due to the existence of these compounds, among others, camels may be affected by cystic ovarian syndrome, leading to delayed pregnancy [20, 23]. Milanesi et al. [26] have identified the presence of estrogens, specifically 17β-estradiol and estrone, in various parts of *Solanum glaucophyllum*, including the seeds, leaves, flowers, and calli. The concentration of these steroids varied depending on the specific tissue or organ being examined. For instance, 17β-estradiol was detected in all the mentioned tissues, with the highest levels observed in the seeds at 120 ng/kg F.W. On the other hand, estrone was found in the calli and seeds, albeit in much lower quantities (a few ng/kg F.W.), and was not present in the aerial organs. Additionally, Milanesi and Boland [27] have also noted the existence of estrogen-like metabolites in the shoots of tomatoes.

Seasonal variations in steroid levels in plants are influenced by various factors, with growth temperature being a significant contributor. Research by Janeczko et al. [28] highlighted the impact of temperature on androgen levels in wheat, showing a notable decrease in androstenedione content when plants were exposed to colder temperatures. This phenomenon was also observed in other plant species like *Nicotiana tabacum* and *Inula helenium*, albeit with varying concentrations. Interestingly, *Digitalis purpurea* did not exhibit the presence of androstenedione. Additionally, Tarkowská's study [29] on *Tribulus terrestris* revealed the detection of testosterone and androst-4-ene-3, 17-dione within a specific concentration range. These findings underscore the intricate relationship between growth conditions and steroid levels in plants, shedding light on the dynamic nature of plant physiology in response to environmental cues. In **Table 1**, Janeczko [20] has presented the presence of estrogens

Plants	Steroids	Content
Populus tremuloides	17β-estradiol	14 pg/g F.W. × 10^{-1} in a bisexual tree (branch 1, November) 2624 pg/g F.W. × 10^{-1} in the reproductive buds of a bisexual tree (March)
Kiwifruit	17β-estradiol	up to 4,000,000 pg/g pollen (dependent on stage of germination)
Kiwifruit	Testosterone	0–2,500,000 pg/g pollen (dependent on stage of germination)
Lettuce, pumpkin, potato, carrot, citrus, apple	17β-estradiol	1300–2200 pg/g F.W.
Pumpkin, potato, carrot, citrus, apple	Estrone	Less than 800 pg/g F.W.
Cakile arabica *Cyperus conglomerates*	Testosterone	3690 pg/g D.W. 2970 pg/g D.W.
Lactuca serriola *Eruca sativa* *Heliotropium bacciferum*	17β-estradiol	379 pg/g D.W. 247 pg/g D.W. 229 pg/g D.W.
Solanum glaucophyllum	17β-estradiol	120 pg/g F.W. (seeds) 4–10 pg/g F.W. (calli, leaves, flowers)
Solanum glaucophyllum	Estrone	3–6 ng/kg F.W. (calli and seeds)
Winter wheat	Androstenedione	6215 pg/g F.W. (leaves of seedlings growing at 20°C)
Nicotiana tabacum *Inula helenium*	Androstenedione	2177 pg/g F.W. (leaves) 3202 pg/g F.W. (leaves)

Table 1.
Presence of estrogens and androgens in plants (F.W.: fresh weight; D.W.: dry weight) [20].

and androgens in plants over the 20 years leading up to 2021; definitely, the highest concentrations of androgen and estrogen were found in pollen.

Steroid hormones have long been associated with the endocrinology of animals, leading to reluctance to acknowledge their presence in higher plants, particularly in the case of testosterone (4-androsten-17-ol-3-one; TS) and its derivatives. This hesitance may stem from the common perception that the effects of steroid hormones are exclusive to animal physiology. However, emerging research suggests that these hormones play a significant role in plant biology as well.

TS, along with epitestosterone and androstenedione, was first isolated from plant sources in 1971. The researchers utilized Scotch pine *Pinus silvestris* pollen and later found these substances, along with progesterone (PRG), in *Pinus nigra* pollen [29]. Pine trees have been identified as a significant source of testosterone, a hormone that plays a crucial role in various physiological functions. Research has shown that testosterone is present in species such as *Pinus tabulaeformis* and *Pinus bungeana*, as well as in the reproductive organs of other plants like ginkgo and lily [30]. Some literature suggests that testosterone and dihydro-testosterone are present in 20 species, such as *Zea mays*, *Hordeum vulgare*, and *Rheum rhabarbarum* [29]. Additionally, Hartmann et al. [31] discussed the normal presence of these phytohormones in diet, highlighting the occurrence of testosterone in *Solanum tuberosum*, *Glycine max*, *Phaseolus vulgaris*, and *Triticum aestivum*, with amounts ranging from 0.02 to 0.2 μg kg^{-1}. The researchers also noted the presence of this androgen in native oils used in human nutrition, such as olive oil, corn oil, and safflower seed oil. Safflower seeds have relatively high phytosterol content, ranging from 2000 to 4500 μg g^{-1}, with β-sitosterol constituting the majority (50–70%) of the total amount of plant sterol [20, 32].

From a biological perspective, the synthesis and biochemical role of testosterone in plants appear to mirror that in animals [29]. This C_{19} steroid is produced through the MVA pathway in the cytosol of plant cells from cholesterol, through a series of enzymatic reactions. These reactions involve the breakdown of the cholesterol side chain into the C21 steroid pregnenolone, then its conversion to androstenedione, and ultimately to TS (**Figure 4**). The conversion to TS was validated through experiments involving feeding 14C-androstenedione, which was transformed into TS in pea and cucumber seedlings, as well as in cultured cells of *Nicotiana tabacum* [29]. Unlike in the animal realm, where TS and other androgens function solely as sex hormones, research has indicated that in plants, they influence not only reproductive development (particularly flowering and floral sex determination) but also vegetative growth [1, 29].

Some literature reported the endogenous formation of weak androgenic substances, such as Boldenone and boldione, from phytosterols in plants. These substances may be produced naturally in plants [33]. Androsta-1,4-diene-3,17-dione (ADD) and androst-4-ene-3,17-dione (AED) are intently correlated compounds. Plant sources containing AED and/or ADD have been identified, with AED found in pine pollen of *Pinus sylvestris* (0.59 μg g^{-1}) and *Pinus nigra* (0.08 μg g^{-1}) as early as 1971, 1979, and 1983 [29]. In 1998, notable levels of AED were also detected in wheat (0.48 ng g^{-1}) and potato (0.05 ng g^{-1}) [31]. Additionally, trace amounts were observed in soybeans, haricot beans, mushrooms, olive oil, safflower oil, wine, and beer. AED was also found in tobacco (Nicotiana tabacum; 2.20 ng g^{-1} F.W.) and elfdock (*Inula helenium*; 3.20 ng g^{-1} F.W.) [33]. Furthermore, AED, ADD, PRG, and TS were conclusively identified in *Tribulus terrestris* [29]. Endogenous steroidal estrogen levels peak

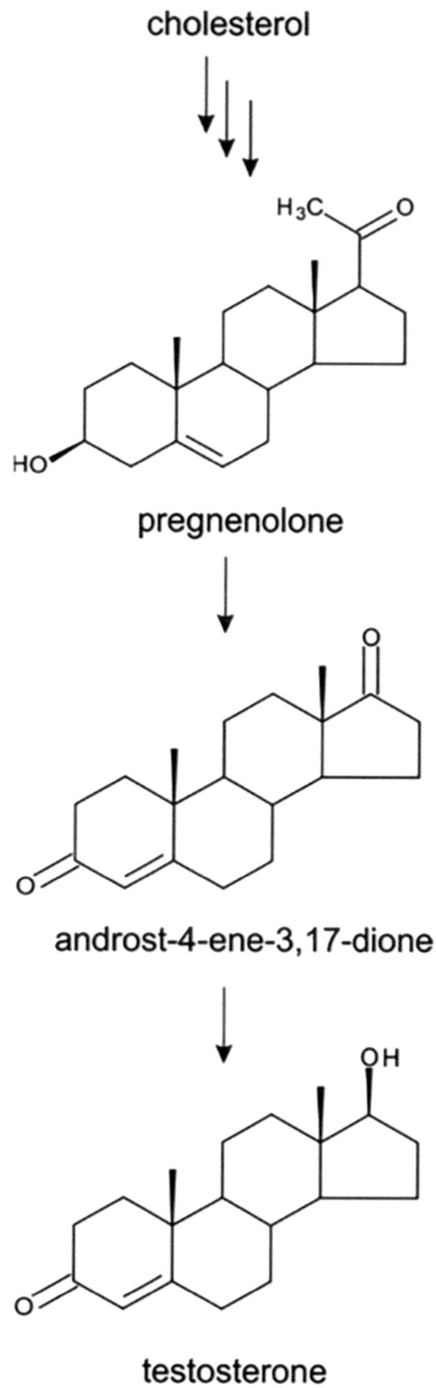

Figure 4.
A simplified biosynthetic pathway of testosterone in plants [29].

in reproductive plant parts like flowers, pollen, fruits, and seeds, while vegetative organs (stem, leaves, roots) have lower concentrations [29, 34]. Estrogens were found in 50% of the 128 species tested, indicating their widespread presence in nature [3].

4. Progesterone in plants

Progesterone, a vital gonadal steroid hormone crucial for the maintenance of early pregnancy and various reproductive processes in mammals, has been found in diverse sources such as false rubber tree shoots and apple seeds [35]. While C21 pregnane steroidal hormones play pivotal roles in mammalian reproductive functions and hormone synthesis, there is a scarcity of information about these compounds in phytochemical literature. The discovery of progesterone in plants [3] showcases how a well-known compound can be identified in natural sources, even in trace amounts, without being previously isolated [36]. Progesterone (PRG) is a C-21 steroid (pregn-4-ene-3, 20-dione).

Progesterone regulates pregnancy progression and menstruation in humans, in addition to serving as a precursor for androgen (C19) and estrogen (C18) production. It also functions as a crucial neurosteroid for brain activities [37]. Studies have revealed the presence of progesterone in various plant species, with levels varying between species and different plant organs. The concentration of progesterone in plant tissues generally remains around 1 μg or less per kg of fresh weight. Research

Plants	**Organ**	**PRG amount (ng kg^{-1} F.W.)**
Dicotyledons		
Thale cress	Foliage	160
	Flowers	400
Pea	Foliage	190
	Root	260
	Ripe seed	410
Common bean	Etiolated seedling	48
Mung bean	Etiolated seedling	21
Tomato	Leaves	25
	Unripe tomato	280
	Red tomato	6
Potato	Tuber	25
Apple	Flesh	150
	Seed	430
Monocotyledons		
Rice	Foliage	1540
	Ear	440
Onion	Bulb	68

Table 2.
Endogenous amounts of PRG in several plants [35].

has identified progesterone in a wide array of plant organs, including shoots, roots, tubers, inflorescences, and seeds, with reproductive tissues containing higher levels of the hormone. Furthermore, genome DNA databases of higher plants have indicated the existence of genes similar to mammalian progesterone-binding proteins, with membrane steroid binding protein (MSBP1) identified in Arabidopsis as a negative regulator of cell elongation [35, 38]. Progesterone has been detected not only in animal-derived products like meat and eggs but also in plant-based foods such as wheat meal, steamed potatoes, and various oils. Simons and Grinwich [3] noted the presence of PRG in a range of plant species (80% of plants from 50 families). Progesterone is naturally present in wheat seedlings in its conjugate form (as glycosides) [38]. According to Iino et al. [35], progesterone was detected in a variety of dicot and monocot species by GC/MS (**Table 2**).

Shiko et al. [39] believed that progestogens and androgens are widespread steroids within the plant kingdom. Several researches utilizing 3H and 14C-labeled precursors have indicated that sitosterol, a prevalent sterol in higher plants, along with the less common sterol cholesterol, can act as precursors of progesterone in plants [29, 40]. Some research also proposes that campesterol and stigmasterol (C_{29}, i.e., 24-ethyl $\Delta^{5,22}$ sterol) could potentially serve as precursors of PRG. The majority of these experiments involve the exogenous application of PRG to various plant systems, such as seedlings or plant cell cultures of different plant species. These studies suggest that PRG plays a role in regulating plant growth and development, impacting both vegetative and generative processes. For example, studies on the model plant *Arabidopsis thaliana* [35] and *Helianthus annuus* have shown that PRG can influence shoot and root growth in a dose-dependent manner [29].

5. Physiological effects of steroids on plants

Brassinosteroids, as highlighted in various studies, play a crucial role in regulating cell growth and differentiation at nano- to micro-molar concentrations. They exhibit diverse regulatory activities such as stimulating cell enlargement and division, inducing leaf bending at joints, altering membrane potentials, regulating gene expression, and influencing nucleic acid and protein metabolism. Notably, these compounds have shown significant promise as plant growth regulators in agriculture [41, 42]. The physiological effects of brassinosteroids are manifold, with exogenous application leading to a wide array of changes in plants. These effects are thought to occur through two main pathways: direct action on the genome and an extra-genetic route, both involving secondary messengers. Studies have demonstrated that brassinosteroids can promote elongation of plant stems when applied externally, with radiolabeling experiments suggesting their movement from roots to shoots via the xylem [42, 43]. Furthermore, research on brassinosteroid-deficient mutants has shed light on the role of these compounds in signal transduction and light-regulated plant development. Mutants such as BRI1, identified through studies on *Arabidopsis*, have provided insights into the molecular mechanisms underlying brassinosteroid responses. The discovery of BRI1's homology to leucine-rich receptor kinases has further deepened our understanding of how brassinosteroids function in plants [44, 45].

The impact of mammalian sex hormones on callus induction has been documented to have various effects. These include the promotion of epinasty, an increase in sugar and protein content, stimulation of reproductive growth and flowering, enhancement of flower number, modulation of the ratio of female to male flowers, as well as improvements in pollination and fertilization processes [1, 46]. The study conducted by Ahmadi-Lashaki et al. [47] found that the application of progesterone did not have a specific effect on the physiological and growth traits of *Petunia hybrida*, *Tagetes erecta*, and *Calendula officinalis*. Despite the potential benefits of progesterone in other plant species, the results of this study suggest that its application may not be effective in enhancing the growth and development of these particular plants. The growth-promoting activity of progesterone was much lower than brassinolide as shown by Li et al. [48].

Recent studies have shed light on the growth-promoting effects of estrone and 17b-estradiol on dwarf pea plants (var. Cud Kelwedonu). Interestingly, it has been discovered that while estrone had a positive impact on mutants and wild-type plants, 17b-estradiol was found to be inactive in both cases. This finding raises questions about the mechanisms by which these hormones exert their effects in plants. It is known that in mammals, progesterone can be converted to estrogens, which then trigger biological responses. However, the results of this study suggest that progesterone may have biological activity in plants even without being transformed into estrogens [35].

Several studies have demonstrated the involvement of brassinosteroids in light-mediated plant development, suggesting a potential mediating role in phytochrome regulatory functions [42, 49, 50]. Additionally, steroids have shown efficacy in enhancing plant resistance against various stressors such as chilling, pathogens, herbicides, and saline condition [51]. Recent findings have highlighted the significant impact of brassinosteroids on modulating plant immunity [42]. Research by Filek et al. [52] revealed that PRG binds to protein receptors in cell membranes, thereby enhancing wheat's tolerance to chilling. Furthermore, the work of Shpakovski et al. [53] emphasized the fundamental interplay between steroid biosynthesis and regulatory systems in both plants and animals. Notably, studies have successfully elevated endogenous progesterone levels in transgenic tobacco and tomato leaves, resulting in positive hormonal effects on plant growth, development, and stress tolerance. Moreover, Pauli et al. [36] definitively identified the presence of PRG in Persian walnut and discovered five other mammalian-type steroids in *Adonis aleppica*.

An interesting impact of MSH is its ability to improve plant resistance to various abiotic stresses [54]. Erdal and Dumlupinar [55] reported that mammal sex hormones (MSHs) mitigate the adverse effects of salinity stress by enhancing the activity of antioxidant enzymes, including SOD, POX, and CAT, as well as increasing proline content. Research has also demonstrated that MSH treatment can stimulate antioxidant process and biosynthesis reactions, leading to a reduction in reactive oxygen species (ROS) in chickpea seedlings [56]. Studies have indicated that the application of PRG and salicylic acid (SA), either individually or in combination, can enhance nutrient (N, Ca, K) uptake and improve plant resilience against injurious elements like Cl and Na in salinity-affected plants [51]. While grasses can still be cultivated in saline conditions, their growth and development may be hindered. However, the adverse effects can be significantly alleviated through the use of PRG, SA, and their mixture [51, 57]. Brassinosteroids have the ability to counteract the inhibitory effects of salinity on seedling growth in groundnut [58]. 24-epibrassinolide and 28-homobrassinolide also alleviated the stress of saline condition and improved *Oriza sativa* germination in saline conditions [59]. Seed treatment with very dilute solutions of BRs has shown significant improvements in the growth of *Oriza* seedlings under salinity [42, 59].

Brassinosteroids have been found to possess stress-protective properties against heavy metals, with 24-epibrassinolide demonstrating a reduction in heavy metal uptake in mustard. When applied to wheat seeds under environmental stress, epibrassinolide led to enhanced germination rates and increased protein content by 15–30%, albeit with a decrease in starch content by 6–19%. Among the two methods of brassinosteroid application, soaking seeds proved more effective than spraying plants. Additionally, brassinolide treating of rice plants was effective in mitigating injury caused by certain herbicides. Studies on oxidative lipid degradation in pea plants indicated that 24-epibrassinolide not only reduced breakdown product levels in normally aerated tissue but also under conditions of hypoxia and elevated CO_2 levels. Compared to kinetin, 24-epibrassinolide treatment was established to be more efficient in various aspects [42].

Immunomodulation is a manner for modifying the immune response that involves inhibiting or modulating the roles of specific antigens in vivo through the intracellular ectopic expression of particular antibodies. This modulation occurs through the interaction of antibodies and antigens, leading to the formation of antigen-antibody complexes. The modulatory impacts of BRs in thale cress seeds highlight their significant function in plant immunomodulation. The less explored trait of immunomodulation by BRs, when administered in precise amounts, has paved the way for new avenues in research on plant growth regulation. Furthermore, it holds the potential for the development of environmentally friendly substitutes for conventional pesticides that are both harmless and biodegradable [42].

Brassinosteroids have demonstrated a practical utility in augmenting the yield of ornamental plants. Significant improvements have been noted particularly in the yield and quality of bulbs and bulbils. Moreover, the application of BRs has been found to boost crop productivity in potatoes, leading to enhanced starch and vitamin C levels in the produce. Additionally, the foliar application of epibrassinolide during the budding or flowering phases has been observed to reduce the susceptibility of plants to fungal infections [42, 60].

The impact of exogenously applied mammal sex hormones (MSH) on plant growth stages, from germination to flowering, has been a subject of research interest [1, 56, 61]. Numerous studies have explored the effects of MSH on various morphological and biochemical parameters, including root and shoot length, enzyme activities, protein, sugar, nucleic acid, and chlorophyll content. These investigations have highlighted the significant stimulation of plant growth and development by MSH, particularly at low concentrations. Elements play crucial roles in the metabolic activities of living organisms, serving structural, electrochemical, and catalytic functions. They are essential for the formation of organic substances and maintaining ion balances, as well as contributing to enzyme formation [61]. Limited studies, such as those by Dogra and Thukral [62, 63] on wheat and maize plants, have examined changes in inorganic constituents like N, P, Fe, Na, and K following MSH application. Additionally, Erdal et al. [64] have reported alterations in inorganic element concentrations in germinating chickpea seeds exposed to progesterone and estradiol.

The impact of various hormones on the growth of sunflower and tomato seedlings has been a subject of recent research. In sunflower seedlings, 17β-estradiol and progesterone at specific concentrations have shown to affect shoot and root growth differently. While they promoted shoot growth, they inhibited root growth, except for progesterone at a lower concentration which actually promoted root elongation. Testosterone, on the other hand, facilitated cotyledon axillary bud formation at certain concentrations [1]. In tomato seedlings, estrone and 17β-estradiol, when administered as sulphate derivatives in the nutrient solution, led to reduced root growth and root number in shoot cuttings. Interestingly, in *Medicago sativa* L., watering with nutrient solutions containing estrone and 17β-estradiol had varying effects depending on the concentrations used. Lower concentrations favored growth and increased dry weight of shoots and roots, whereas higher concentrations inhibited plant growth. The authors highlighted the potential impact of estrogen levels found in sewage water on the vegetative growth of alfalfa plants. Recent data also suggest that estrogens and progesterone can stimulate winter wheat seedling roots and leaves when grown in vitro, but higher concentrations of these steroids can lead to a slight inhibition in seedling growth [1, 65].

Bonner et al. [66] conducted a study using a steroid biosynthesis inhibitor (SK & F7997) to halt the blossoming progression in an SD plant rough cocklebur. However, this compound also interfered with the production of membrane sterols. In non-vernalized plants of chicory, flowering was induced by estrone and 17β-estradiol, with 55 and 85% of plants flowering, respectively, while control plants remained in a vegetative state. Androgens like TS were found to be ineffective in reproductive development in scarlet sage [67]. In a separate experiment by Biswas et al. [68], androstane and androsterone did not promote flowering in chrysanths.

The application of exogenous progesterone significantly affects plant shoot and root growth, seed germination, and reproductive development (**Figure 5**). Progesterone, a hormone primarily associated with female reproductive functions in animals, shares striking similarities with plant hormones in terms of its role in mediating growth and development processes, as well as regulating responses to environmental stresses. While progesterone is not traditionally classified as a plant hormone, its functions parallel those of known plant hormones such as auxins, cytokinins, and abscisic acid. Plant hormones play a crucial role in coordinating various physiological processes in plants, including seed germination, root and shoot growth, flowering, and fruit development. Similarly, progesterone has been found to

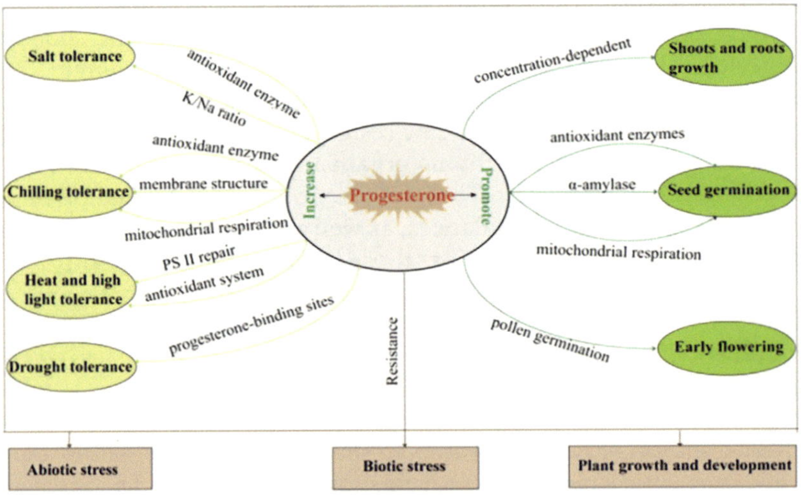

Figure 5.
The summary of plant progesterone regulation during growth, development, and biotic/abiotic stress responses [69].

influence cell division, elongation, and differentiation in animal cells, suggesting a conserved mechanism of action across kingdoms. Furthermore, both plant hormones and progesterone are involved in regulating responses to biotic and abiotic stresses. Plant hormones help plants adapt to challenging environmental conditions such as drought, salinity, and pathogen attacks. Similarly, progesterone has been shown to modulate immune responses and stress tolerance in animals and plants, indicating a shared function in enhancing resilience to adverse conditions. In conclusion, although progesterone is not officially recognized as a plant hormone, its functional similarities with plant hormones highlight the interconnectedness of biological processes across different organisms [69].

Li et al. [69] fully summarized the regulation of progesterone on plant growth and development and the alleviating effects of progesterone on biotic and abiotic stresses in plants in two (**Tables 3** and **4**).

Türkoğlu et al. [91] studied the effect of different mammalian sex hormones (17 β-estradiol, estrogen, progesterone, and testosterone) in several concentrations on genetic or epigenetic levels in bean plants and found that genetic strength is decreased. It was found that the CRED-iPBS profile highlighted a significant increase in methylation levels associated with DNA cytosine nucleotide when exposed to 10^{-4} mM of estrogen hormone. Notably, polymorphism was evident across all hormone administrations in comparison to the control group (without hormone), signifying a reduction in genomic stability at higher concentrations. These findings collectively suggest that 17 β-estradiol, estrogen, progesterone, and testosterone impact genomic stability in bean plants, leading to epigenetic modifications that play a crucial role in regulating gene expression.

Plant growth and development	Progesterone (PRG) role	Plants	Ref
Foliage and root growth	PRG controlled plant growth in a dosage-related manner.	Thale cress	[35]
		Sunflower	[70]
		Chickpea	[55]
Tissue culture	PRG enhanced foliage and callus production.	Sainfoin	[71]
	PRG regulated responded embryogenic callus and regenerable callus induction.	Wheat	[72]
Seed germination	PRG improved seed germination.	Chickpea	[54]
		Common bean	[56]
		Maize	[73, 74]
Generative progress	PRG augmented increasingly with pollen germination.	Kiwifruit	[22]
	PRG enhanced pollen germination and tube enlargement.	Tobacco	[75, 76]
	PRG encouraged plant flowering and induced generative growth.	Wheat	[77, 78]
		Thale cress	[79]

Table 3.
The effects of PRG on plant life process [69].

Biotic/abiotic stress	Progesterone role	Plants	Ref
Salt	PRG induced enzymatic and non-enzymatic antioxidant systems and improved the amounts of osmoprotectants.	Wheat	[80]
	PRG increased SOD, POX, and CAT actions and alleviated the salt-reduced K/Na ratio.	Bean	[54]
	PRG improved antioxidant activity and osmoprotectant accumulation.	Maize	[81]
	PRG enhanced salinity tolerance and augmented pigments and antioxidant enzyme activities.	Kentucky bluegrass	[82]
Chilling	PRG stimulated relative leaf water content, chlorophyll content, and antioxidative activity.	Chickpea	[83]
	PRG stimulated the mitochondrial respiratory pathway and upregulated the transcript level and protein accumulation of alternative oxidase (AOX).	Maize	[84]
	PRG encouraged AOX and enhanced enzyme and non-enzymatic antioxidant protection systems.	Dwarf banana	[85]
	PRG improved the transcription level of IbAOX1 and the activity of AOX, prevented the creation of chilling damage, decreased membrane penetrability, MDL and ROS levels, and improved the antioxidant defenses.	Sweet potato	[86]
	The increase in area per lipid molecule by PRG led to the formation of more flexible surface structures in monolayers.	Wheat	[52]
Drought	Drought caused to increase PRG-binding sites on the cell membrane of Katoda (drought-sensitive cultivar) but not in Monsun (drought-tolerant cultivar), while this stress caused to augment of PRG-binding sites in the cytoplasm of Monsun, but not in Katoda.	Wheat	[87]
	More-expressing animals' CYP11A1 in *Solanum lycopersicum* can considerably improve tolerance to water deficit and prolonged dehydration.	Tomato	[53]
High temperature and high irradiance	PRG improved overheating-induced H_2O_2, MDA, and ionic leakage, increased the production of SOD, CAT, POX, and reduced photosystem II damage by stimulating D1 protein phosphorylation.	Wheat	[88]
	PRG improved antioxidant resistance system and simplified D1 protein strength under temperature and high irradiance stress.	Wheat	[89]
Biological stresses	PRG reduced the necrosis and the ion leakage, and enhanced the efficacy of PSII affected by pseudomonad	Thale cress	[90]
	CYP11A1-overexpressing transgenic tobacco exhibited resistance to contamination by fungal pathogens *Botrytis cinerea.*	Tobacco	[53]

Table 4.
The positive properties of progesterone (PRG) on environmental stresses in plants [69].

6. Conclusions

Numerous studies have been conducted to investigate the impact of steroid hormones on the growth and development of plants. The findings have revealed that steroid sex hormones, including progesterone, estrone, beta-estradiol, and testosterone, play a significant role in stimulating growth and development, callus development, cell division and elongation of roots and stems, and enhancing pollination in plants. Moreover, these hormones have been found to have a positive effect on plant stress response. Steroid hormones are considered secondary metabolites that are synthesized under specific conditions, such as exposure to stress. Among these compounds, progesterone has been shown to enhance the antioxidant properties of plants, thereby aiding them in coping with environmental challenges. Overall, the research suggests that steroid hormones can have beneficial effects on plant physiology and resilience.

Acknowledgements

The authors would like to thank colleagues for their assistance.

Conflict of interest

The authors have no conflict of interest to declare.

Notes/thanks/other declarations

This research received no external funding.

Author details

Shahram Sedaghathoor*, Seyedeh Khadijeh Abbasnia Zare and Ali Shirinpur-Valadi
Department of Horticultural Science, Rasht Branch, Islamic Azad University, Rasht, Iran

*Address all correspondence to: sedaghathoor@yahoo.com

References

[1] Janeczko A, Skocczowski A. Mammalian sex hormones in plants. Folia Histochemica Et Cytobilogica. 2005;**43**(2):71-79. DOI: 10.5603/4616

[2] Dohrn M, Faure W, Poll H, Blotevogel W. Tokokinine, Stoff mit sexualhormonartiger Wirkung aus Pflanzenzellen. Medizinische Klinik. 1926;**22**:1417-1419

[3] Simons RG, Grinwich DL. Immunoreactive detection of four mammalian steroids in plants. Canadian Journal of Botany. 1989;**67**:288-296. DOI: 10.1139/b89-042

[4] Dogra R, Thukral AK. Effect of pre-sowing treatment of steroid hormones on proteins, nucleic acids and some enzymes in wheat plants. Journal of Indian Botanical Society. 1996;**75**:125-128

[5] Kaur A, Thukral AK. Animal hormones and plant growth and development. In: Dhir KK, Sareen TS, editors. Frontiers in Plant Science Research. Delhi: Bhagwati Enterprises; 1993. pp. 271-297

[6] Wang HJ, Wei ZY, Li J, Wang XL. Brassinosteroids. In: Li JY, Li CY, Smith SM, editors. Hormone Metabolism and Signaling in Plants. Cambridge: Academic Press; 2017. pp. 291-326

[7] Bajguz A, Chmur M, Gruszka D. Comprehensive overview of the Brassinosteroid biosynthesis pathways: Substrates, products, inhibitors, and connections. Frontiers in Plant Science. 2020;**11**:1034. DOI: 10.3389/fpls.2020.01034

[8] Bajguz A. Brassinosteroids in microalgae: Application for growth improvement and protection against abiotic stresses. In: Hayat S, Yusuf M, Bhardwaj R, Bajguz A, editors. Brassinosteroids: Plant Growth and Development. Singapore: Springer; 2019. pp. 45-58

[9] Nolan TM, Vukašinović N, Liu D, Russinova E, Yin Y. Brassinosteroids: Multidimensional regulators of plant growth, development, and stress responses. Plant Cell. 2020;**32**:295-318. DOI: 10.1105/tpc.19.00335

[10] Sakurai A. Brassinosteroid biosynthesis. Plant Physiology and Biochemistry. 1999;**37**:351-361

[11] Asami T, Nakano T, Fujioka S. Plant brassinosteroid hormones. Vitamins & Hormones. 2005;**72**:479-504

[12] Fujioka S, Sakurai A. Brassinosteroids. Natural Product Reports. 1997;**14**:1-10

[13] Ohnishi T. Recent advances in brassinosteroid biosynthetic pathway: Insight into novel brassinosteroid shortcut pathway. Journal of Pesticide Science. 2018;**43**(3):159-167. DOI: 10.1584/jpestics.D18-040

[14] Nelson D, Werck-Reichhart D. A P450-centric view of plant evolution. The Plant Journal. 2011;**66**(1):194-211

[15] Guengerich FP, Munro AW. Unusual cytochrome P450 enzymes and reactions. Journal of Biological Chemistry. 2013;**288**(24):17065-17073

[16] Asami T, Yoshida S. Brassinosteroid biosynthesis inhibitors. Trends in Plant Science. 1999;**4**:348-353

[17] Asami T, Nakano T, Nakashita H, Sekimata K, Shimada Y, Yoshida S. The

influence of chemical genetics on plant science: Shedding light on functions and mechanism of action of brassinosteroids using biosynthesis inhibitors. Journal of Plant Growth Regulation. 2003;**22**:336-349

[18] Rozhon W, Akter S, Fernandez A, Poppenberger B. Inhibitors of brassinosteroid biosynthesis and signal transduction. Molecules. 2019;**24**:4372. DOI: 10.3390/molecules24234372

[19] Simerský R, Novák O, Morris DA, Pouzar V, Strnad M. Identification and quantification of several mammalian steroid hormones in plants by UPLC-MS/MS. Journal of Plant Growth Regulation. 2009;**28**:125-136. DOI: 10.1007/s00344-009-9081-z

[20] Janeczko A. Estrogens and androgens in plants: The last 20 years of studies. Plants. 2021;**10**(12):2783. DOI: 10.3390/plants10122783

[21] Khaleel TF, Dillman R, Gretch D. Estradiol distribution during the development and expression of reproductive structures in *Populus tremuloides* Michx. Sexual Plant Reproduction. 2003;**16**:35-42. DOI: 10.1007/s00497-003-0171-y

[22] Speranza A, Crosti P, Malerba M, Stocchi O, Scoccianti V. The environmental endocrine disruptor, Bisphenol A, affects germination, elicits stress response and alters steroid hormone production in kiwifruit pollen. Plant Biology. 2011;**13**:209-217. DOI: 10.1111/j.1438-8677.2010.00330.x

[23] Zeitoun M, Alsoqeer AR. Detection of sex steroid hormones in alfalfa and some rangeland native species in Saudi Arabia and their subsequent effects on camel reproduction. Global Vets. 2014;**13**:33-38. DOI: 10.5829/idosi.gv.2014.13.01.84119

[24] Lu J, Wu J, Stoffella PJ, Wilson PC. Analysis of bisphenol A, nonylphenol, and natural estrogens in vegetables and fruits using gas chromatography–tandem mass spectrometry. Journal of Agricultural and Food Chemistry. 2013;**61**(1):84-89. DOI: 10.1021/jf304971k

[25] Palacios OM, Cortes HN, Jenks BH, Maki KC. Naturally occurring hormones in foods and potential health effects. Toxicology Research and Application. 2020;**4**:2397847320936281. DOI: 10.1177/2397847320936281

[26] Milanesi L, Monje P, Boland R. Presence of estrogens and estrogen receptor-like proteins in *Solanum glaucophyllum*. Biochemical and Biophysical Research Communications. 2001;**289**:1175-1179. DOI: 10.1006/bbrc.2001.6079

[27] Milanesi L, Boland R. Presence of estrogen receptor (ER)-like proteins and endogenous ligands for ER in solanaceae. Plant Science. 2004;**166**:397-404

[28] Janeczko A, Biesaga-Kościelniak J, Dziurka M, Filek M, Hura K, Jurczyk B, et al. Biochemical and physicochemical background of mammalian androgen activity in winter wheat exposed to low temperature. Journal of Plant Growth Regulation. 2018;**2018**(37):199-219. DOI: 10.1007/s00344-017-9719-1

[29] Tarkowská D. Plants are capable of synthesizing animal steroid hormones. Molecules. 2019;**24**(14):2585. DOI: 10.3390/molecules24142585

[30] ZhongHan Y, Yin T, ZongXun C. Changes of the contents of testosterone-steroidal sex hormone in reproductive organs of *Lilium davidii* Duch. Acta Botanica Sinica. 1994;**36**:215-220

[31] Hartmann S, Lacorn M, Steinhart H. Natural occurrence of steroid

hormones in food. Food Chemistry. 1998;**62**(1):7-20. DOI: 10.1016/S0308-8146(97)00150-7

[32] Hall C III. Overview of the oilseed safflower (*Carthamus tinctorius* L.). Reference Module Food Science. 2016. DOI: 10.1016/B978-0-08-100596-5.00030-5

[33] Poelmans S, De Wasch K, Martelé Y, Schilt R, Van Hoof N, Noppe H, et al. The Possible Transformation of Phytosterols to Boldenone. Proceedings Euro Food Chem XII: Strategies for Safe Food; 2003. pp. 24-26

[34] Sláma K. Development and metamorphosis in invertebrates–hormonal control. General and Comparative Endocrinology. 1980;**40**:313-314

[35] Iino M, Nomura T, Tamaki Y, Yamada Y, Yoneyama K, Takeuchi Y, et al. Progesterone: Its occurrence in plants and involvement in plant growth. Phytochemistry. 2007;**68**(12):1664-1673. DOI: 10.1016/j.phytochem.2007.04.002

[36] Pauli GF, Friesen JB, Gödecke T, Farnsworth NR, Glodny B. Occurrence of progesterone and related animal steroids in two higher plants. Journal of Natural Products. 2010;**73**(3):338-345. DOI: 10.1021/np9007415

[37] Graham JD, Clarke CL. Physiological action of progesterone in target tissues. Endocrine Reviews. 1997;**18**(4):502-519

[38] Janeczko A. The presence and activity of progesterone in the plant kingdom. Steroids. 2012;**77**(3):169-173. DOI: 10.1016/j.steroids.2011.10.012

[39] Shiko G, Paulmann MJ, Feistel F, Ntefidou M, Hermann-Ene V, Vetter W, et al. Occurrence and conversion of progestogens and androgens are conserved in land plants. New Phytologist. 2023;**240**(1):318-337

[40] Lindemann P, Luckner M. Biosynthesis of pregnane derivatives in somatic embryos of digitalis lanata. Phytochemistry. 1997;**46**(3):507-513. DOI: 10.1016/S0031-9422(97)00315-4

[41] Clouse SD, Sasse JM. Brassinosteroids: Essential regulators of plant growth and development. Annual Review of Plant Biology. 1998;**49**:427-451. DOI: 10.1146/annurev.arplant.49.1.427

[42] Bhardwaj R, Arora HK, Nagar PK, Thukral AK. Brassinosteroids—A novel group of plant hormones. In: Trivedi PC, editor. Plant Molecular Physiology. Jaipur: Aavishkar Publishers; 2006. pp. 58-84

[43] Fujioka S, Sakurai A. Biosynthesis and metabolism of brassinosteroids. Physiologia Plantarum. 1997;**100**:710-715. DOI: 10.1111/j.1399-3054.1997.tb03078.x

[44] Clouse SD, Langford M, McMorris TC. A brassinosteroid-insesitive mutant in Arabidopsis thaliana exhibits multiple defects in growth and development. Plant Physiology. 1996;**111**:671-678. DOI: 10.1104/pp.111.3.671

[45] Szekeres M, Nemeth K, Kalman ZK, et al. Brassinosteroids rescue the deficiency of CYP90, a cytochrome P450, controlling cell elongation and de-etiolation in Arabidopsis. Cell. 1996;**85**:171-182. DOI: 10.1016/s0092-8674(00)81094-6

[46] Sedaghathoor S, Zakibakhsh-Mohammadi P. Effect of time of application and amounts of mammalian sex hormone progesterone and gibberellic acid on the growth

of Zinnia elegans. Revista Chapingo. Serie horticultura. 2019;**25**(1):61-73. DOI: 10.5154/R.RCHSH.2018.08.017

[47] Ahmadi-Lashaki M, Sedaghathoor S, Kalatehjari S, Hashemabadi D. The physiological and growth response of Petunia hybrida, Tagetes erecta, and Calendula officinalis to plant and human steroids. AIMS Agriculture and Food. 2018;**3**(2):85-96. DOI: 10.3934/agrfood.2018.2.85

[48] Li J, Nagpal P, Vitart V, McMorris TC, Chory J. A role for brassinosteroids in light-dependent development of *Arabidopsis*. Science. 1996;**272**:398-401. DOI: 10.1126/science.272.5260.398

[49] Chory J, Li J. Gibberellins, brassinosteroids and light-regulated development. Plant, Cell & Environment. 1997;**20**:801-806. DOI: 10.1046/j.1365-3040.1997.d01-99.x

[50] Karnachuk RA, Golovatskaya IF, Efimova MV, Khripach VA. Action of epibrassinolide on morphogenesis and hormonal balance in Arabidopsis seedlings at green light. Russian Journal of Plant Physiology. 2002;**49**(4):530-533. DOI: 10.1023/A:1016372228174

[51] Sabzmeydani E, Sedaghathoor S, Hashemabadi D. Progesterone and salicylic acid elevate tolerance of *Poa pratensis* to salinity stress. Russian Journal of Plant Physiology. 2020;**67**:285-293. DOI: 10.1134/S1021443720020132

[52] Filek M, Rudolphi-Skórska E, Sieprawska A, Kvasnica M, Janeczko A. Regulation of the membrane structure by brassinosteroids and progesterone in winter wheat seedlings exposed to low temperature. Steroids. 2017;**128**:37-45. DOI: 10.1016/j.steroids.2017.10.002

[53] Shpakovski GV, Spivak SG, Berdichevets IN, Babak OG, Kubrak SV, Kilchevsky AV, et al. A key enzyme of animal steroidogenesis can function in plants enhancing their immunity and accelerating the processes of growth and development. BMC Plant Biology. 2017;**17**(Suppl. 1):120-131. DOI: 10.1186/s12870-017-1123-2

[54] Erdal S, Genisel M, Turk H, Gorcek Z. Effects of progesterone application on antioxidant enzyme activities and K^+/Na^+ ratio in bean seeds exposed to salt stress. Toxicology and Industrial Health. 2012;**28**(10):942-946. DOI: 10.1177/0748233711430975

[55] Erdal S, Dumlupinar R. Mammalian sex hormones stimulate antioxidant system and enhance growth of chickpea plants. Acta Physiologiae Plantarum. 2011;**33**(3):1011-1017. DOI: 10.1007/s11738-010-0634-3

[56] Erdal S, Dumlupinar R. Progesterone and β-estradiol stimulate seed germination in chickpea by causing important changes in biochemical parameters. Zeitschrift für Naturforschung C. 2010;**65**(3-4):239-244. DOI: 10.1515/znc-2010-3-412

[57] Sabzmeydani E, Sedaghathoor S, Hashemabadi D. Salinity response of Kentucky bluegrass (*Poa pratensis* L.) as influenced by salicylic acid and progesterone. Revista Chapingo. Serie Horticultura. 2020;**26**(1):49-63. DOI: 10.5154/r.rchsh.2019.08.012

[58] Vardhini BV, Anjum NA. Brassinosteroids make plant life easier under abiotic stresses mainly by modulating major components of antioxidant defense system. Frontiers in Environmental Science. 2015;**2**:67. DOI: 10.3389/fenvs.2014.00067

[59] Anuradha S, Rao SSR. Effect of brassinosteroids on salinity stress induced inhibition of seed

germination and seedling growth of rice (*Oryza sativa* L.). Plant Growth Regulation. 2001;**33**:151-153. DOI: 10.1023/A:1017590108484

[60] Khripach V, Zhabinskii V, de Groot A. Twenty years of brassinosteroids: Steroidal plant hormones warrant better crops for the XXI century. Annals of Botany. 2000;**86**:441-447. DOI: 10.1006/anbo.2000.1227

[61] Erdal S, Dumlupinar R. Exogenously treated mammalian sex hormones affect inorganic constituents of plants. Biological Trace Element Research. 2011;**143**(1):500-506. DOI: 10.1007/s12011-010-8857-0

[62] Dogra R, Thukral AK. Effect of steroid on some inorganic constituents of wheat plants. Current Research Plant Science. 1996;**2**:155-160

[63] Dogra R, Thukral AK. Effect of Steroids on Inorganic Constituents of Maize Leaves. Jodhpur: Environment and Development. Scientific Publishers; 1998. pp. 269-273

[64] Erdal S, Dumlupinar R, Cakmak T, Taskin M. Determination of some inorganic element concentration changes in germinating chickpea seeds exposed to progesterone and β-estradiol by using WDXRF spectroscopic technique. Fresenius Environmental Bulletin. 2010;**19**:507-515

[65] Shore LS, Kapulnik Y, Ben-Dor B, Fridman Y, Wininger S, Shemesh M. Effects of estrone and 17β-estradiol on vegetative growth of Medicago sativa. Physiologia Plantarum. 1992;**84**:217-222

[66] Bonner J, Heftmann E, Zeevaart JA. Suppression of floral induction by inhibitors of steroid biosynthesis. Plant Physiology. 1963;**38**(1):81-88. DOI: 10.1104/pp.38.1.81

[67] Kopcewicz J. Influence of estrogens on flower formation in Cichorium intybus L. Naturwissenschaften. 1970;**57**(3):136-136. DOI: 10.1007/BF00600070

[68] Biswas PK, Paul KB, Henderson JHM. Effects of steroids on chrysanthemum in relation to growth and flowering. Nature. 1967;**213**(5079):917-918. DOI: 10.1038/213917a0

[69] Li H, Chen L, Chen H, Xue R, Wang Y, Song J. The role of plant progesterone in regulating growth, development, and biotic/abiotic stress responses. International Journal of Molecular Sciences. 2022;**23**(18):10945. DOI: 10.3390%2Fijms231810945

[70] Bhattacharya B, Gupta K. Steroid hormone effects on growth and apical dominance of sunflower. Phytochemistry. 1981;**20**:989-991. DOI: 10.1016/0031-9422(81)83014-2

[71] Dadaşoğlu E, Tosun M. The effect of mammalian sex hormones on in vitro properties of sainfoin (*Onobrychis sativa* L.) Fresenius environ. Bullet. 2018;**27**:7222-7229

[72] Turkoglu A. Effects of mammalian sex hormones on regeneration capacity, retrotransposon polymorphism and genomic instability in wheat (*Triticum aestivum* L.). Plant Cell Tissue and Organ Culture. 2023;**152**:647-659. DOI: 10.1007/s11240-022-02440-z

[73] Erdal S, Dumlupinar R, Cakmak T, Genisel M. Mammalian sex hormones influence germination velocity and enzyme activities in germinating maize seeds. Fresenius Environmental Bulletin. 2010;**19**:1458-1465

[74] Turk H. Progesterone promotes mitochondrial respiration at the biochemical and molecular level in germinating maize seeds. Plants. 2021;**10**:1326. DOI: 10.3390/plants10071326

[75] Ylstra B, Touraev A, Brinkmann AO, Heberle-Bors E, Tunen A. Steroid hormones stimulate germination and tube growth of in vitro matured tobacco pollen. Plant Physiology. 1995;**107**:639-643. DOI: 10.1104/pp.107.2.639

[76] Spivak S, Berdichevets I, Yarmolinsky D, Maneshina T, Shpakovski G, Kartel N. Construction and characteristics of transgenic tobacco *Nicotiana tabacum* L. plants expressing CYP11A1 cDNA encoding cytochrome P450SCC. Russian Journal of Genetics. 2009;**45**:1067-1073. DOI: 10.1134/S1022795409090075

[77] Janeczko A, Filek W. Stimulation of generative development in partly vernalized winter wheat by animal sex hormones. Acta Physiologiae Plantarum. 2002;**24**:291-295. DOI: 10.1007/s11738-002-0054-0

[78] Janeczko A, Oklestkova J, Novak O, Śniegowska-Świerk K, Snaczke Z, Pociecha E. Disturbances in production of progesterone and their implications in plant studies. Steroids. 2015;**96**:153-163. DOI: 10.1016/j.steroids.2015.01.025

[79] Janeczko A, Filek W, Biesaga-Kościelniak J, Marcińska I, Janeczko Z. The influence of animal sex hormones on the induction of flowering in *Arabidopsis thaliana*: Comparison with the effect of 24-epibrassinolide. Plant Cell, Tissue and Organ Culture. 2003;**72**:147-151. DOI: 10.1023/A:1022291718398

[80] Erdal S. Alleviation of salt stress in wheat seedlings by mammalian sex hormones. Journal of the Science of Food and Agriculture. 2012;**92**:1411-1416. DOI: 10.1002/jsfa.4716

[81] Erdal S. Exogenous mammalian sex hormones mitigate inhibition in growth by enhancing antioxidant activity and synthesis reactions in germinating maize seeds under salt stress. Journal of the Science of Food and Agriculture. 2012;**92**:839-843. DOI: 10.1002/jsfa.4655

[82] Sabzmeydani E, Sedaghathoor S, Hashemabadi D. Effect of salicylic acid and progesterone on physiological characteristics of Kentucky bluegrass under salinity stress. Revista Ciencias Agrícolas. 2021;**38**:111-124. DOI: 10.22267/rcia.213801.151

[83] Genisel M, Turk H, Erdal S. Exogenous progesterone application protects chickpea seedlings against chilling-induced oxidative stress. Acta Physiologiae Plantarum. 2013;**35**:241-251. DOI: 10.1007/s11738-012-1070-3

[84] Erdal S, Genisel M. The property of progesterone to mitigate cold stress in maize is linked to a modulation of the mitochondrial respiratory pathway. Theoretical and Experimental Plant Physiology. 2016;**28**:385-393. DOI: 10.1007/s40626-016-0076-4

[85] Hao J, Li X, Xu G, Huo Y, Yang H. Exogenous progesterone treatment alleviates chilling injury in postharvest banana fruit associated with induction of alternative oxidase and antioxidant defense. Food Chemistry. 2019;**286**:329-337. DOI: 10.1016/j.foodchem.2019.02.027

[86] Chen H, Zhou S, Li X, Yang H. Exogenous progesterone alleviates chilling injury by upregulating IbAOX1 to mediate redox homeostasis and proline accumulation in postharvest sweet potato tuberous root. Postharvest Biology

and Technology. 2022;**183**:111738. DOI: 10.1016/j.postharvbio.2021.111738

[87] Janeczko A, Oklešťková J, Siwek A, Dziurka M, Pociecha E, Kocurek M, et al. Endogenous progesterone and its cellular binding sites in wheat exposed to drought stress. The Journal of Steroid Biochemistry and Molecular Biology. 2013;**138**:384-394. DOI: 10.1016/j.jsbmb.2013.07.014

[88] Xue R, Wang S, Xu H, Zhang P, Li H, Zhao H. Progesterone increases photochemical efficiency of photosystem II in wheat under heat stress by facilitating D1 protein phosphorylation. Photosynthetica. 2017;**55**:664-670. DOI: 10.1007/s11099-016-0681-0

[89] Su X, Wu S, Yang L, Xue R, Li H, Wang Y, et al. Exogenous progesterone alleviates heat and high light stress-induced inactivation of photosystem II in wheat by enhancing antioxidant defense and D1 protein stability. Plant Growth Regulation. 2014;**74**:311-318. DOI: 10.1007/s10725-014-9920-1

[90] Janeczko A, Tóbiás I, Skoczowski A, Dubert F, Gullner G, Barna B. Progesterone moderates damage in Arabidopsis thaliana caused by infection with *Pseudomonas syringae* or *P. fluorescens*. Plantarum. 2013;**57**:169-173. DOI: 10.1007/s10535-012-0142-y

[91] Türkoğlu A, Haliloğlu K, Balpinar Ö, Öztürk HI, Özkan G, Poczai P. The effect of mammalian sex hormones on polymorphism and genomic instability in the common bean (*Phaseolus vulgaris* L.). Plants. 2022;**11**(15):2071. DOI: 10.3390/plants11152071

Chapter 3

Progestin Selectivity in Clinical Applications

Hisham Arab

Abstract

This chapter presents a thorough examination of synthetic progestins in obstetric and gynecologic practice, highlighting their specific use in several clinical scenarios, including miscarriage, luteal phase support, menstrual problems, and endometriosis. Drawing from existing literature, the chapter explores the specific biological, pharmacological, and clinical characteristics of progestins -especially dydrogesterone -emphasizing their subtle functions in different reproductive health conditions. The study primarily revolves around dydrogesterone, with a thorough investigation that includes data extracted from the literature on its molecular structure, *in vitro* and *in vivo* findings, clinical data obtained from randomized clinical trials, and systematic reviews. This chapter intends to provide the reader with a detailed understanding of the distinct clinical applications and differential selectivity of synthetic progestins, with a particular focus on the unique features of dydrogesterone. The goal is to equip the reader with a nuanced comprehension of these drugs. This resource is beneficial for healthcare practitioners, researchers, and academicians who want a more detailed understanding of the complex relationship between synthetic progestins and reproductive health in different clinical situations.

Keywords: progestin, miscarriage, pregnancy, menstrual, dydrogesterone

1. Introduction

1.1 A refresher on progesterone

Progesterone, one of the first hormones to be discovered, is a 21-carbon sex steroid produced from cholesterol by the conversion of pregnenolone [1, 2]. Progesterone is primarily synthesized in the corpus luteum of the ovaries and also by the placenta [1, 2]. Progesterone derives its name from its role as a hormone essential for initiating and maintaining pregnancy. It is referred to as progestational, combining the prefix "pro," meaning "for," with the root "gest," meaning "pregnancy" [3].

Although that would mean that progesterone is the key physiological component in the reproductive system, it can also modulate neurotransmitter systems, including the serotonergic, cholinergic, and dopaminergic systems, in addition to immunomodulatory effects [1]. Progesterone also has significant functions in other non-reproductive organs, including the mammary gland for lactation preparation, the circulatory system, the central nervous system, and the bones [4]. Natural or P4 progesterone is vital in pregnancy from conception to delivery. It also has clinical uses in the treatment of preterm labor, miscarriage, and infertility [5]. Progesterone can be utilized to cause amenorrhea or regular bleeding, sub-atrophy, or pre-decidual alterations by adjusting the dosage, duration of treatment, and method of administration [3].

More recent research has enhanced our comprehension of the inhibitory effects of progesterone on immune responses, specifically inflammatory responses. The activation of dendritic cells, macrophages, and natural killer (NK) cells in mice is inhibited by progesterone. The administration of progesterone to rat dendritic cells stimulated with lipopolysaccharide inhibits the synthesis of interleukin (IL)-1 and tumor necrosis factor (TNF)-α, both of which are pro-inflammatory cytokines. Progesterone inhibits the secretion of the cytokine IL-12, which stimulates T-cell activation. Many of these inhibitory effects are achieved through the inhibition of NF-kB activation. It has been documented that progesterone, besides impeding cytokine production, also inhibits the synthesis of chemokines, including RANTES and macrophage inflammatory protein-1β, by CD8+ T lymphocytes. Progesterone exerts intriguing immunoregulatory effects through its ability to modulate the differentiation of various immune cell subpopulations [6].

Throughout the early 2000s, researchers became particularly interested in investigating the involvement of progesterone in both genomic (nuclear) and non-genomic (extranuclear) receptor pathways. These mechanisms work together to directly impact cells and tissues. Due to its lipophilic nature, progesterone easily passes through cell membranes via diffusion. It then interacts with progesterone receptor A (PR-A) and progesterone receptor B (PR-B) at the nuclear level. This interaction triggers the activation of approximately 300 co-regulators, which act on ribosomal RNA. As a result, corresponding proteins are produced. Nuclear progesterone receptors (nPR) require a time span of minutes or hours to initiate ribosomal transcription and serve as the primary controllers of female reproductive processes. The genomic receptors PR-B and PR-A have overlapping regions in the DNA binding domain and the ligand binding domain, but they have distinct amino acid sequences. Specifically, PR-A has 164 fewer amino acids than PR-B. In humans, cells expressing PR-B and PR-A are equally prevalent under normal physiological conditions. Nevertheless, myometrial tissue has a significant amount of a third isoform of nPR, known as PR-C [4].

Progesterone has a key role in facilitating crosstalk between various uterus and placenta cells, influencing many biological processes. Progesterone regulates the process of decidualization by governing the development of endometrial stromal cells. If this signaling is disrupted, it can result in pregnancy difficulties such as recurrent miscarriage and pre-eclampsia. This highlights the critical role of progesterone in this communication between cells. The release of progesterone by the ovaries induces the creation of activin A by cells in the lining of the uterus, which in turn affects the attachment of the embryo's outer layer to the uterine wall. Progesterone is recognized as a crucial factor in promoting cellular modifications that support an embryo's attachment and the placenta's development. Although the endocrinological functions of progesterone have been extensively studied in the past, its involvement in communication with immune cells in the placenta has been evident in recent times [6].

Before we move on to progestins. The difference between "progestins" and "progestogens" is worth highlighting. Progestogens are substances that exhibit progestational action. They encompass both artificial progestogens and organic progesterone, also referred to as P4. In contrast to natural P4, synthetic progestins such as dydrogesterone do not possess tranquilizing, antiandrogenic, diuretic, tocolytic, or neuroprotective properties. These effects are potentially significant for supporting pregnancy from conception to delivery [7]. While the term progestin refers only to synthetic progestational agents that have been synthesized to replicate the activity of P4 [8].

1.2 A quick overview of progestins

The early advancement in steroid hormone bioengineering involved the elimination of the 19-carbon from natural progesterone to create a more powerful synthetic progestational agent. Several novel progestins have been created after the introduction of norethindrone and norethynodrel. The overall objective is to produce chemicals with enhanced potency, specifically targeting the ovary and the endometrium, while ensuring increased safety and control over the menstrual cycle. Additionally, the aim is to minimize adverse effects and provide acceptable non-contraceptive advantages. Progestin molecules exhibit varying affinities for the progesterone receptor, androgen receptor, estrogen receptor, glucocorticoid receptor, and mineralocorticoid receptor. At present, the contraceptive progestins that are accessible are either derived from natural testosterone or progesterone [9].

Progestins can be classified into various categories, including retroprogesterone (e.g., dydrogesterone) and progesterone derivatives (e.g., medrogestone). The compounds mentioned are multiple derivatives of 17alpha-hydroxyprogesterone, 19-norprogesterone, 19-nortestosterone, and spironolactone. Examples of these derivatives include chlormadinone acetate, cyproterone acetate, medroxyprogesterone acetate, megestrol acetate, nomegestrol, promegestone, trimegestone, nesterone, norethisterone (NET), lynestrenol, levonorgestrel, desogestrel, gestodene, norgestimate, dienogest, and drospirenone (**Figure 1**) [10]. The progestins within the same class have distinct biological activities compared to each other. Thus, analyzing progestins individually, rather than grouping them by class, may provide the most valuable understanding of their specific effects [11].

Progestins, including progesterone (P4), exert their effects through the binding with progesterone receptors (PRs), which exist in two isoforms (A and B) resulting from a single gene located on chromosome 11. These isoforms exhibit distinct tissue

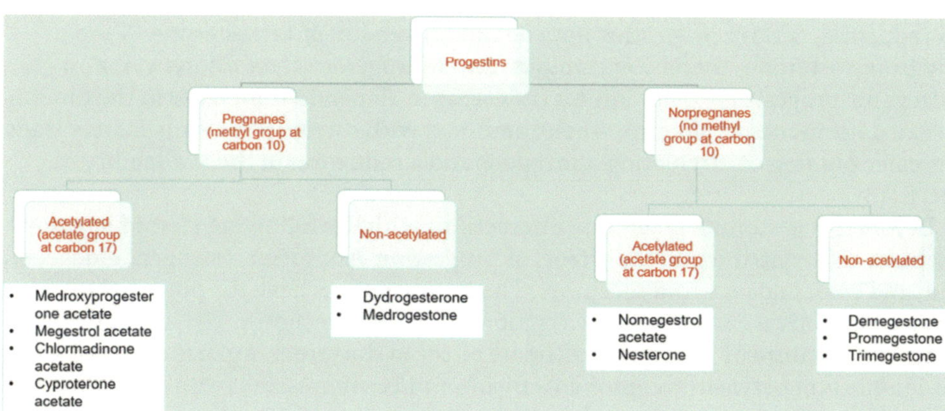

Figure 1.
Classification of progestins that are structurally related to progesterone.

distributions and functions. The structural composition of PR includes a DNA-binding domain, zinc fingers, a hinge region, and a ligand-binding domain. Genomic interactions occur when P4 binds to the ligand-binding site, forming progesterone response elements (PREs) and a transcriptional complex that modulates gene expression within minutes to hours. Notably, a third isoform (PR C) has been identified, primarily expressed in myometrial cells, lacking a DNA binding domain but capable of binding to progesterone. Evidence suggests that PR C may inhibit other isoforms by sequestering available progesterone. Isoform A dominates when PR A and B are coexpressed in the same tissue. Moreover, PRs interact with various receptors, such as estrogen receptor, androgen receptor, glucocorticoid receptor, and mineralocorticoid receptor, displaying agonistic or antagonistic effects through specific interactions. The involvement of coactivators or corepressors further adds complexity to the regulatory mechanisms governing PR-mediated actions. Overall, these insights highlight the intricate structural and functional aspects of PRs, contributing to our understanding of progestins' diverse and nuanced actions [12].

The effectiveness of progestins is primarily categorized by three distinct actions, which are the primary acts that enable progestins to be beneficial in various circumstances [13]. The following items are included:

1. Progestational activity refers to the capacity to induce the transformation of the endometrium into the secretory phase and sustain a pregnancy.

2. Exhibiting anti-estrogenic activity: The capability to reduce the expression of estrogen receptors and subsequently diminish the thickness of the endometrium stimulated by estrogen.

3. Antiandrogenic activity refers to the capability of inhibiting the binding of testosterone (T) to androgen receptors, hence reducing the impact of androgens and counteracting the action of 5α-reductase.

The biological effects of progestogens are contingent upon the presence of estrogens, particularly in most tissues, as the expression of progesterone receptors (PR) is reliant on their presence. However, progestogens suppress the expression of estrogen receptors [14, 15].

By competitively inhibiting the androgen receptor or binding to the enzyme 5-α reductase, certain progestins impede the conversion of testosterone (T) to dihydrotestosterone, thereby exerting an antiandrogenic effect. Moreover, non-androgenic progestins do not inhibit the estrogen-dependent increase in the binding of sexual hormones to globulin when combined with estrogen. This ultimately leads to greater binding of circulating androgens and a reduction in the availability of free T [13].

Beyond progesterone receptors, interactions with the following steroid hormone receptors also contribute to the effects of progestins: Androgen, estrogen, glucocorticoid, and mineralocorticoid receptors. These interactions have the potential to either trigger transactivation or inhibit activation of a steroid receptor. The agonistic or antagonistic nature of progestin's ultimate effect in the target organ is determined by the equilibrium between receptor coactivators and corepressors recruited by the molecule. While all progestins exert the anticipated effect on the uterine endometrium by binding to the progesterone receptor, their activity profiles in other target tissues are unique and may not be identical among progestins of the same class [16].

Furthermore, the literature showed the anti-inflammatory and immunomodulatory effects of p4 and progestins. Some of the anti-inflammatory and immunomodulatory actions of P4 and its derivatives are associated with the inhibition of NF-kB and COX, the inhibition of prostaglandin synthesis, the regulation of T lymphocytes, the regulation of the production of pro- and anti-inflammatory cytokines, and the phenomenon of immune tolerance. Besides, the inhibition of proliferative signaling pathways and the antagonistic action against estrogen receptor beta-mediated signaling are pro-inflammatory and mitogenic factors. Moreover, steroid receptor cochaperone HSP90 and immunophilins FKBP51 and FKBP52 represent a crucial key in the intracellular signaling of steroid hormones, including progesterone. Thus, due to their combined effect, P4 and progestins could be considered promising alternative steroid hormones to glucocorticoids in the treatment of inflammatory diseases, including endometriosis, stress-related disorders, rheumatoid arthritis, and miscarriages, especially hormone-resistant chronic inflammatory diseases [17].

Anti-estrogenic effects of progestogens and progestin in the endometrium are attributed to the activation of 17β-Hydroxysteroid dehydrogenase type 2, which catalyzes the conversion of estradiol to estrone, and estrone sulfotransferase, which promotes conjugation of estrone; these effects include a decrease in ER expression [12].

Progestins have clinical uses thanks to their therapeutic applications and because their bioavailability and half-lives are superior to P4. Currently, a multitude of additional characteristics of these agents has been elucidated, enabling their utilization in diverse therapeutic contexts—including contraception, hormonal replacement therapy (HRT), and the management of gynecological ailments such as endometriosis and polycystic ovary syndrome [18]. However, progestins have various effects according to their interactions with receptors, including AR, GR, and MR. These interactions can lead to side effects such as acne, hyperlipidemia, salt and water retention, and bloating. Additionally, progestins typically function as an antagonist of MR, resulting in lower water retention and weight [13, 19].

2. Dydrogesterone: molecular structure and characteristics

Dydrogesterone can be considered a stereoisomer of progesterone, with a slight difference in its molecular structure. In dydrogesterone, the hydrogen atom at carbon 9 is positioned in the β position, while the methyl group at carbon 10 is in the α position. This arrangement is the opposite of the structure found in progesterone, leading to its designation as "retro" progesterone. Furthermore, a double bond is present between carbon 6 and 7, altering the flat steroid configuration and resulting in a "bent" conformation that exhibits increased rigidity compared to progesterone. It is believed that this explains why dydrogesterone is highly selective for progesterone receptors, displaying strong progestogenic effects while lacking any significant agonistic effects on androgen, glucocorticoid, and mineralocorticoid receptors. When comparing progesterone and dydrogesterone, it is worth noting that dydrogesterone has a higher oral bioavailability. This, combined with its strong affinity for progesterone receptors and its effectiveness at a low dose, may help to reduce the occurrence of side effects [20].

The molecular structure of this compound bears a striking resemblance to natural progesterone (**Figure 2**), yet it exhibits improved oral bioavailability. Dydrogesterone and progesterone have distinct structural features that set them apart. With its inverted configuration at C9 and C10 and an additional C6-C7 double bond, dydrogesterone exhibits a bent shape geometry. In contrast, progesterone has an almost planar geometry [21].

Early endocrinological studies in animal models indicated that dydrogesterone exhibited significant progestogenic effects while lacking androgenic, glucocorticoid, or estrogenic activity. Dydrogesterone is often regarded as more potent than progesterone, as noted in the lower milligram dose needed to achieve comparable efficacy in comparison to micronized vaginal progesterone (MVP) [22].

Studies conducted *in vitro* revealed that dydrogesterone did not exhibit any significant agonistic effects on androgen, glucocorticoid, and mineralocorticoid receptors. On the other hand, progesterone exhibited important agonistic activity at androgen receptors while showing little to no agonist activity at glucocorticoid or mineralocorticoid receptors. It was found that dydrogesterone exhibited lower antagonistic activity at glucocorticoid and mineralocorticoid receptors when compared to progesterone. In addition, it is worth noting that progesterone demonstrated significant antiandrogenic effects at the pre-receptor level, effectively inhibiting over 90% of 5α-reductase type 2, which is an enzyme responsible for androgen production. On the other hand, dydrogesterone and 20α-dihydro dydrogesterone (DHD) exhibited comparatively weaker inhibition of this enzyme, reaching only up to 16%. The data presented here collectively illustrates the high selectivity of dydrogesterone for progesterone receptors compared to progesterone. Additionally, dydrogesterone exhibits minimal antiandrogenic effects at the pre-receptor level, thereby reducing other receptors' activation and undesirable effects [23].

Dydrogesterone functions by offering progesterone-like support during the luteal phase of the menstrual cycle. By imitating the actions of natural progesterone, dydrogesterone enhances the vital processes during this stage, including promoting decidualization and developing a receptive endometrial lining. The actions described foster an environment that supports the successful implantation of embryos and the maintenance of early pregnancy [24].

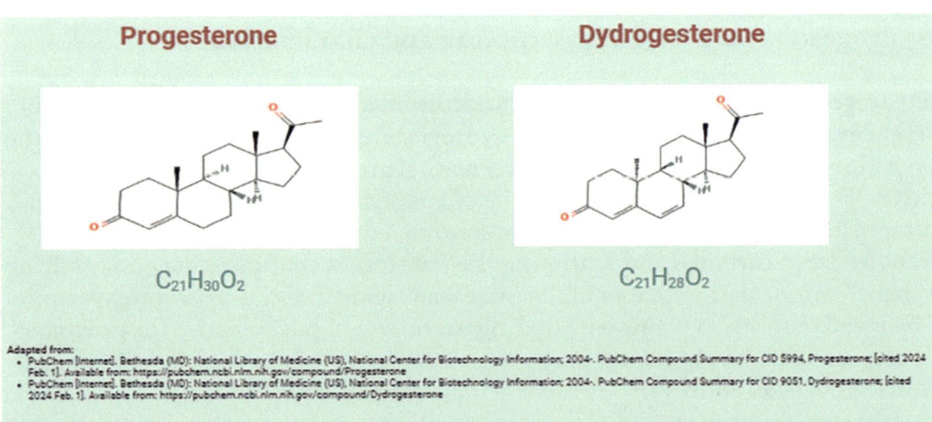

Figure 2.
Comparison between the chemical structure of dydrogesterone and progesterone. Adapted from PubChem [Internet]. Bethesda (MD): National Library of medicine (US), National Center for biotechnology information; 2004; PubChem compound summary for CID 5994, progesterone; [cited 2024 Feb. 1]. Available from: https://pubchem.ncbi.nlm.nih.gov/compound/Progesterone; PubChem [Internet]. Bethesda (MD): National Library of medicine (US), National Center for biotechnology information; 2004-. PubChem compound summary for CID 9051, Dydrogesterone; [cited 2024 Feb. 1]. Available from: https://pubchem.ncbi.nlm.nih.gov/compound/Dydrogesterone

The retro-structure and the C6-C7 double bond of dydrogesterone provide it with a distinct advantage. These features cause the molecule to adopt a rigid conformation well-suited for binding with the PR. Dydrogesterone's enhanced rigidity contributes to its selectivity, unlike natural progesterone, which exhibits less selectivity due to its ability to bind to various receptors in different conformations. Due to its enhanced bioavailability and the progestational activity of its main metabolites (20-, 21- and 16-hydroxy derivatives), dydrogesterone requires a significantly lower equivalent dose compared to oral or vaginal micronized progesterone [10].

As shown in **Table 1**, dydrogesterone is highly selective for progesterone receptors due to its unique structure [10, 23, 25].

Dydrogesterone is quickly taken up by the body and fully broken down through metabolism. Following oral administration, the levels of dydrogesterone and its main metabolite, 20-dihydro dydrogesterone (DHD), in the plasma peak after 0.5–2.5 hours. Interestingly, the concentration of DHD in the plasma is significantly greater than that of the parent drug. The elimination half-lives of dydrogesterone and DHD are 5–7 and 14–17 hours, respectively. Dydrogesterone does not have any clinically significant pharmacokinetic interactions. Preclinical studies have shown that dydrogesterone has no mutagenic, teratogenic, or carcinogenic effects. Additionally, pharmacovigilance data has not found any evidence of congenital malformations linked to the use of dydrogesterone during pregnancy [26].

3. Clinical applications of dydrogesterone

Dydrogesterone has been widely available in numerous countries for over six decades to address progesterone deficiency and its related conditions. These include irregular cycles, dysfunctional uterine bleeding, dysmenorrhea, endometriosis, secondary amenorrhea, premenstrual syndrome, threatened and habitual miscarriage, infertility due to luteal insufficiency, and hormone replacement therapy. Extensive research and pharmacovigilance data have not found any evidence of dydrogesterone being teratogenic or carcinogenic, nor have they linked its use during pregnancy to congenital malformations (**Figure 3**) [27].

Biological activity [a]	Dydrogesterone	Progesterone
Progestogenic	+	+
Anti-gonadotropin	—	+
Anti-estrogenic	+	+
Estrogenic	—	—
Androgenic	—	—
Antiandrogenic	± [b]	±
Glucocorticoid	—	+
Anti-mineralocorticoid	±	+

[a] *Therapeutic dosage.*
[b] *Dydrogesterone demonstrates less antiandrogenic effects than progesterone.*
DYD –dydrogesterone, PR-A -progesterone receptor A; + "efficacious"; ± "less efficacious"; – "not efficacious".

Table 1.
A comparison between the biological activities of dydrogesterone and progesterone.

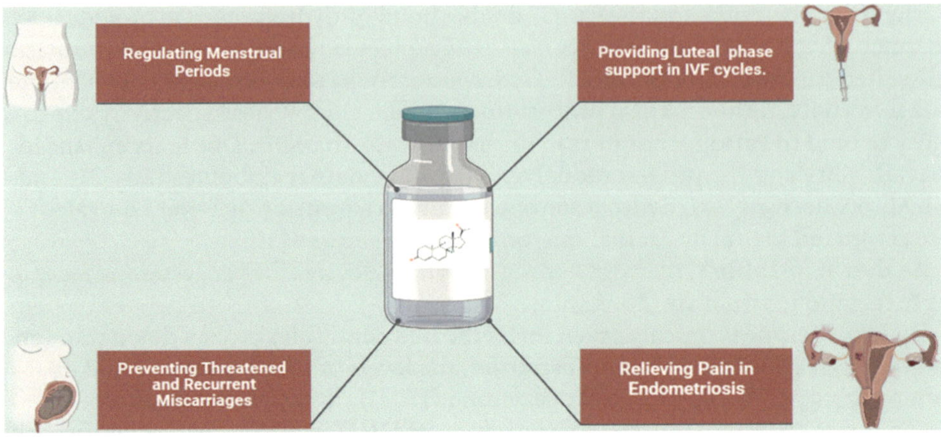

Figure 3.
Some clinical applications of dydrogesterone.

3.1 Preventing threatened and recurrent miscarriages

Several randomized controlled trials have demonstrated that women who were at risk of early pregnancy loss and received dydrogesterone experienced significantly lower rates of miscarriage compared to those who received bed rest with or without supportive care [28–30].

According to a systematic review, dydrogesterone was found to significantly decrease the odds of miscarriage by 47% compared to standard care. Additionally, it was associated with an absolute decrease of 11% in the miscarriage rate [31].

This has been supported by a study that highlighted that the occurrence of miscarriage in patients suffering from bleeding in the first trimester was notably lower in the group that received total progesterone compared to the control group. The percentage of miscarriage in the total progesterone group was 13.0%, while in the control group it was 21.7%. The odds ratio was calculated to be 0.53, with a 95% confidence interval of 0.36 to 0.78. The statistical analysis showed a significant difference between the two groups, with a p-value of 0.001 and an I2 value of 0%. In addition, the occurrence of miscarriage showed a substantial decrease in the group receiving oral dydrogesterone compared to the control group (11.7% versus 22.6%; odds ratio, 0.43; 95% CI, 0.26 to 0.71; P = 0.001; I2, 0%). Similarly, the vaginal progesterone group also exhibited a lower rate of miscarriage compared to the control group, although this difference was not statistically significant (15.4 versus 20.3%; odds ratio, 0.72; 95% CI, 0.39 to 1.34; P = 0.30; I2, 0%). Nevertheless, there was no discernible difference in the occurrence of miscarriage between the groups receiving oral dydrogesterone and vaginal progesterone. Progesterone therapy, particularly oral dydrogesterone, is highly effective in preventing miscarriage in pregnant women who are facing the risk of abortion [32].

Another systematic review assessing ten studies examining the effects of progestins versus placebo has concluded a statistically significant decrease in the pregnancy loss rates in patients treated with progestins, including dydrogesterone [33].

These results are supported by another randomized controlled trial that examined the effectiveness of dydrogesterone versus vaginal progesterone in women with recurrent pregnancy loss (RPL) and presenting with first-trimester bleeding. The study revealed that patients treated with dydrogesterone experienced a faster cessation of bleeding compared to those treated with vaginal progesterone [34].

In a recent meta-analysis, Zhao et al., conducted a comprehensive assessment of the effectiveness and safety of different progestogens. They analyzed data from 59 randomized controlled trials involving a total of 10,424 women. The study concluded that oral dydrogesterone was more effective than vaginal progesterone in treating threatened miscarriages [35].

Based on the previous data, it is no wonder that dydrogesterone has been recommended for the management of early pregnancy loss by multiple international guidelines, including the European Progestin Club (EPC), European Society of Human Reproduction and Embryology (ESHRE), Royal Australian and New Zealand College of Obstetricians and Gynecologists (RANZCOG), German (DGGG), Austrian (OEGGG), and Swiss (SGGG) Societies of Gynecology and Obstetrics, National Institute for Health and Care Excellence (NICE), and Russian Society of Obstetricians and Gynecologists. Miscarriage in addition to local guidelines in Saudi Arabia, Malaysia, China, Vietnam, Taiwan, Indonesia, Mexico, and the Philippines [36].

3.2 Regulating menstrual periods

Research demonstrated the efficacy of dydrogesterone as a therapeutic agent for the management of dysfunctional uterine hemorrhage. The utilization of this technique has prevented patients from undergoing hysterectomy, hence reducing their exposure to the potential risks associated with general anesthesia and surgery. Additionally, it has alleviated the strain and fiscal burden on the hospital, staff, and the state [37].

A multicenter study involving 104 women was done to evaluate the effects of cyclical dydrogesterone, which is commonly used for estrogen replacement therapy. The trial was double-masked, randomized, and placebo-controlled. Secondary amenorrhea is the medical term used to describe the stopping of menstrual periods after they have already started. Nevertheless, it has been precisely delineated by many definitions, some of which coincide with oligomenorrhea (scanty menstrual flow occurring at intervals of 35 days to 6 months). This indicates the broad range of patients affected by this disorder. The approximate prevalence of secondary amenorrhea in women of reproductive age is approximately 3%. Ultimately, dydrogesterone is markedly more effective than a placebo in stimulating the occurrence of withdrawal bleeding and sustaining regular menstrual bleeding in women who have secondary amenorrhea and possess normal levels of estrogen [38].

A pilot randomized controlled trial revealed that dydrogesterone was equally effective to vaginal micronized progesterone in the treatment of dysfunctional uterine bleeding [39].

A multicenter observational study involving 210 women diagnosed with heavy menstrual bleeding (HMB) aimed to investigate the impact of dydrogesterone treatment on health-related quality of life (HRQoL). Women with a pictorial blood assessment chart (PBAC) score exceeding 100 were considered to have HMB. After administration of dydrogesterone for three consecutive cycles, participants were assessed using the 5-dimensional EuroQol (EQ-5D) for HRQoL, PBAC score, and menstrual cycle diaries at entry (visit 2) and the end of each treatment cycle (visits 3 to 5). A notable decrease in PBAC score indicated that improved severity of menstruation was reported. Additionally, menstrual flow assessments shifted toward medium and light categories, with only six women describing their flow as heavy post-treatment compared to 201 before treatment. Dydrogesterone treatment was well-tolerated, with a 14.3% incidence of adverse events, predominantly pallor (3.8%) and anemia (2.4%), which need further hematologic treatment to correct HMB-associated iron deficiency anemia. In conclusion, the study demonstrates that dydrogesterone treatment substantially and significantly enhances HRQoL in women suffering from HMB by effectively addressing the severity of menstrual bleeding [40].

Dydrogesterone, taken as an orally administered retroprogesterone, is commonly employed to address inadequacy in progesterone levels, such as irregularities in the menstrual cycle. A non-interventional, single-arm, post-marketing, observational study was conducted to assess the impact of dydrogesterone on the regularization of the menstrual cycle. It showed that the administration of dydrogesterone resulted in the attainment of menstrual cycle regularization and a decrease in both menstrual pain and anxiety, both throughout the treatment period and the subsequent 6-month observation period [27]. This was further established by a more recent post-marketing study that showed that administering dydrogesterone orally throughout the latter half of the menstrual cycle has demonstrated a reduction in menstrual abnormalities. This study is prospective and observational. Furthermore, dydrogesterone effectively normalizes and enhances the length of the menstrual cycle, diminishes the volume of bleeding, alleviates menstrual discomfort, and prevents the recurrence of irregular cycles up to 6-months following the cessation of treatment [41].

Another literature review examining the efficacy of medicines, the frequency of complications (for example, the risk of venous thromboembolism when taking combined oral contraceptives, depending on the type of progestogen), and contraindications of progestins in the management of abnormal uterine bleeding in postmenopausal women revealed that dydrogesterone therapy has demonstrated great efficacy in restoring regularity to irregular menstrual periods, as evidenced by randomized controlled trials. Dydrogesterone is a drug that does not affect metabolism. It does not have any androgenic, glucocorticoid, mineralocorticoid, or antigonadotropic effects. It does not worsen insulin resistance or dyslipidemic disorders or affect the hemostatic system. Therefore, it can be safely recommended for a broad range of women with abnormal uterine bleeding including adolescents [42].

A single-arm, prospective, non-interventional, observational research was conducted after the product had been marketed. In conclusion, the administration of dydrogesterone therapy proved to be an efficient method for achieving menstrual cycle regularization in Chinese patients with abnormal uterine bleeding. Furthermore, the neutral effects of dydrogesterone on sex hormones, as well as the metabolic level, provide further evidence that it plays a role in the regulation of irregular menstrual cycles [43].

Another study presented an interesting finding. In this study, patients were treated with dydrogesterone, norethisterone acetate (NETA), medroxyprogesterone acetate, or nomegestrol acetate. The main objective was to determine the effects of these four compounds on basal body temperature (BBT), depression, and anxiety. Interestingly, dydrogesterone did not affect BBT like NETA or other progesterones. Furthermore, dydrogesterone reduced anxiety compared to other treatments [44].

3.3 Luteal phase support in IVF cycles

Overall, substantial data indicates that dydrogesterone has a high absorption level when taken orally and a strong affinity for progesterone receptors. A study even suggested it is efficacious at a 10 to 20 times lower dosage than micronized progesterone. Dydrogesterone exhibits a favorable safety and tolerability profile with few adverse effects. Consequently, it is considered an optimal choice for use in assisted reproductive technology (ART) as a luteal phase support (LPS) agent. Oral dydrogesterone is equally beneficial as vaginal progesterone for LPS in women undergoing fresh *in vitro* fertilization (IVF) [45].

Dydrogesterone can also be used as an add-on therapy. Retrospective cohort research that was performed at a single site from 2013 to 2019 revealed that the utilization of dydrogesterone in conjunction with micronized progesterone gel resulted in a greater clinical pregnancy rate and live birth rate compared to the exclusive use of micronized progesterone gel in frozen-thawed embryo transfer (FET) cycles [46].

Another pilot single-masked randomized controlled trial reported that it was effective, and patients tended to prefer oral dydrogesterone due to its ease of use, cheaper cost, and greater efficacy. Therefore, dydrogesterone can be suggested as an alternative to intramuscular or vaginal supplements for LPS in artificial FET cycles [47].

A clinical trial has indicated that oral dydrogesterone (40 mg/day) is as efficacious as vaginal micronized progesterone in terms of clinical outcomes, patient satisfaction, and tolerability for LPS in women undergoing IVF [48].

3.4 Relieving pain in endometriosis

Evidence from 1976 reported that after the administration of 5 mg of dydrogesterone twice daily to 49 endometriosis patients, five patients were asymptomatic following 9-months of treatment. In most cases, subjective symptoms resolved within 4 to 9 weeks; dyspareunia, on average, required more time. A "cure" of endometriosis was verified in 30 out of 32 patients who underwent culdoscopy following one or two courses of treatment. Following treatment, ten of nineteen infertile patients became expectant. Two patients experienced transient mastalgia and vertigo as the only adverse effects. There were no reported cases of amenorrhea or other disruptions of the menstrual cycle [49].

In women with dysmenorrhea, cyclic application of dydrogesterone has also been shown to induce regular menstruation, reduced blood loss, and fewer days of bleeding, in addition to providing exceptional symptomatic relief [50].

The ORCHIDEA study showed that the extended cyclical and uninterrupted courses of dydrogesterone treatment showed significant and comparable decreases in the intensity of long-lasting pelvic discomfort and painful menstruation and resulted in notable enhancements in all aspects of quality of life and sexual satisfaction measured in the study [51].

Compared with gestrinone, dydrogesterone relieved dysmenorrhea, increased the pregnancy rate, and reduced the risk of certain adverse events. Compared with Gonadotropin releasing hormone - agonist (GnRH-a), dydrogesterone also lowered the risk of endometriosis recurrence and elevated transaminase levels.

Dydrogesterone exhibits superior efficacy in alleviating pelvic discomfort and dysmenorrhea compared to gestrinone while also demonstrating a lower incidence of adverse effects. Conceiving while using dydrogesterone may provide a higher level of safety. GnRH agonists exhibit significant adverse effects, including hot flushes, vaginal dryness, headaches, superficial dyspareunia, and a propensity for the emergence of osteoporotic alterations. Moreover, it is advised to refrain from attempting pregnancy while doing this therapy. Dydrogesterone significantly enhances pregnancy rates within the first year following surgery, compared to receiving no treatment. The rise in pregnancy rates becomes statistically significant around the 12-month mark [52]. Dydrogesterone's diverse advantages in alleviating symptoms and improving fertility highlight its attractive position as a treatment for pelvic discomfort and dysmenorrhea, compared to alternative options such as gestrinone and GnRH agonists.

It is worth mentioning that dydrogesterone is not the only progestin used for managing endometriosis. Levonorgestrel, medroxyprogesterone acetate, NETA, dienogest, and dydrogesterone are the most well-known progestogens utilized in endometriosis-affected patients [53]. In 2018, a study was published that examined the therapeutic and side effects, as well as the molecular mechanisms of action, of dydrogesterone and dienogest in mice with endometriosis. After carefully evaluating the size and volume of lesions, histological parameters, and biochemical markers of proliferation and apoptosis throughout and after treatment, it was determined that dydrogesterone and dienogest exhibit efficacy in treating endometriosis. These treatments demonstrate selective effects on proliferation, apoptosis, and the molecular mechanisms associated with endometriosis. It has been observed that both dydrogesterone and dienogest significantly impact the size of lesions and inhibit the growth of cells in endometriotic foci. The primary therapeutic effects of this treatment are associated with progesterone receptors. It works by suppressing cell proliferation and activating apoptosis in endometriotic foci. Nevertheless, the antiproliferative and apoptosis effects were less pronounced in dienogest when compared to dydrogesterone [54]. A study reported that while both had comparable safety profiles, a lower dose of dienogest was more effective than dydrogesterone for relieving pain associated with endometriosis [55]. Given its potent effects on the endometrium, NETA is a useful treatment for endometriosis and endometrial hyperplasia. However, special consideration is needed in cases of high risk for thromboembolic events and when treating women experiencing migraine with aura [56]. On the other hand, there is evidence supporting that dydrogesterone therapy does not increase the risks for venous thromboembolism [57]. Another study reported that dydrogesterone therapy was associated with decreased levels of fibrinogen and Lp(a), hence decreasing the risk for future cardiovascular events [58]. This was further confirmed by a recent literature review reporting that dydrogesterone therapy was associated with minuscule risks for cardiac manifestations and venous thromboembolism [59].

4. Dydrogesterone's safety profile

Dydrogesterone has been commercially available and utilized since the 1960s to address various diseases related to inadequate progesterone levels. It is recommended for treating both threatened and idiopathic recurring miscarriages in multiple nations across the globe. According to the cumulative statistics on dydrogesterone exposure from April 1960 to April 2021, it is predicted that the total patient exposure after the drug was released on the market will be 137.5 million patient treatment years. According to sales data from 2014, it was predicted that around 20 million fetuses were exposed to dydrogesterone in the womb between April 1960 and April 2014. Dydrogesterone was correlated with elevated levels of patient and clinician satisfaction. At the end of treatment (EOT), 89.6% of patients expressed satisfaction or high satisfaction with their treatment, while investigators assessed the overall response to treatment as good or excellent in 85.8% of patients [27].

Dydrogesterone exhibits no estrogenic, androgenic, or adrenocorticoid activity. It cannot be converted into estrogens and only shows anti-estrogenic effects in specific target organs, such as the endometrium. It is worth noting that this synthetic progestational agent has shown promising results, as its endometrial response closely resembles that of natural progesterone. Interestingly, it does not impact the pituitary-adrenal axis, and there is no decrease in plasma progesterone levels when administered after ovulation. In addition, it shows no or only mild suppression of ovulation, which is often seen with other progestogens. Furthermore, it does not impact coagulation, blood lipids, or glucose/insulin parameters. It is also not harmful to the liver and does not lead to a rise in body temperature. It has been observed to have a similar effect on aldosterone as natural progesterone but does not significantly impact water and electrolyte balance. Unlike progesterone, dydrogesterone does not get eliminated as pregnanediol in urine. Thus, it remains feasible to measure urinary pregnanediol as an indicator of natural progesterone secretion in women receiving dydrogesterone treatment [25].

From 1977 to 2005, pharmacovigilance data identified a mere 28 instances of congenital abnormalities that may be associated with fetal exposure to dydrogesterone. The defects exhibited a wide range of variations without any discernible pattern of anomalies. Therefore, there is no evidence of a correlation between congenital abnormalities and the usage of dydrogesterone [26]. A more recent study also supported the previous statement and attributed the safety of taking dydrogesterone during pregnancy to its well-established safety profile [22].

An important note is that dydrogesterone is less likely to cause DNA fragmentation and repair synthesis in primary cultures of rat hepatocytes. A study comparing the three progestogens that include double bonds, namely dydrogesterone, dienogest, and 1,4,6-androstatriene-17-ol-3-one acetate (ADT), and cyproterone acetate revealed that cyproterone acetate exhibited the highest DNA damaging potency, followed by dienogest, ADT, and finally dydrogesterone [60].

Another study revealed that dydrogesterone's high selectivity for progesterone receptors helped to minimize the risk of side effects in women undergoing assisted reproduction. They added that the distinctive molecular arrangement of dydrogesterone enables its effectiveness when taken orally at low therapeutic dosages, so circumventing the tolerability concerns linked to the vaginal administration of progesterone [24]. This may be due to the unique structure of dydrogesterone, which allows efficacy with oral administration at low therapeutic doses, avoiding the tolerability issues associated with vaginal administration of progesterone. In addition, dydrogesterone's high selectivity for progesterone receptors may help to limit the risk of side effects.

Another study examining patients with threatened miscarriage revealed that the incidence of congenital, familial, and genetic diseases was low and comparable across oral dydrogesterone and MVP gel in the Lotus I and II trials and later meta-analyses and subpopulation studies [20, 59, 61–63].

An intriguing hypothesis posits that progesterone may influence bone metabolism. To explore this, we focused on dydrogesterone, a compound closely mirroring the chemical structure of natural progesterone while devoid of any androgenic effects. Our investigation involved a comparative analysis, specifically examining the impact of a daily regimen of dydrogesterone compared to estradiol treatment. Surprisingly, the dydrogesterone regimen led to an increase in osteoclasts, though without a discernible augmentation in their functionality. The work of Roux C. et al. proved that in rat models subjected to ovariectomy, dydrogesterone failed to inhibit bone resorption, and interestingly, it exhibited no influence on the positive effects induced by estradiol. These findings shed light on the complex interplay between dydrogesterone and bone metabolism and the contrasting impact observed compared to estradiol treatment. Further research is warranted to unravel dydrogesterone's nuanced dynamics and potential implications on bone health, offering valuable insights into its specific interactions within the context of bone metabolism regulation [64].

Progesterone is involved in insulin resistance by blocking the PI3-kinase pathway and reducing the expression of insulin receptor substrate 1 (IRS1). Estradiol causes insulin resistance by activating the c-Jun N-terminal kinase (JNK) through the estrogen receptor located on the cell membrane. This leads to the phosphorylation of serine residues on the insulin receptor substrate-1 (IRS-1) [65]. Additionally, some research studies claimed that the use of progestogen supplements during pregnancy to lower the chances of preterm birth can raise the likelihood of developing gestational diabetes mellitus. Conversely, dydrogesterone does not possess diabetogenic properties [66, 67].

5. Conclusions

To summarize, investigating progestogens, particularly dydrogesterone, concerning reproductive health and gynecological problems unveiled a complex and diverse scenario. The ongoing research highlights the intricate nature of women's reproductive health, pregnancy, and the process of maximizing positive pregnancy outcomes. Further research is needed to optimize care to establish a comprehensive therapeutic approach that combines validated psychological support with pharmaceutical techniques. To recognize the importance of patient education in improving treatment adherence and outcomes, it is important to focus on teaching patients about gynecological disorders, pregnancy complications, and pregnancy loss, as well as the advantages of dydrogesterone. In the future, the idea of tailoring treatment to individual patients using prediction models that consider their specific traits and biomarkers has the potential to greatly enhance the effectiveness of dydrogesterone therapies. Moreover, a crucial aspect of future investigation is examining the long-term safety of dydrogesterone and its potential effects on the health of both the mother and the fetus. An in-depth evaluation of its risk-benefit profile over prolonged durations will yield significant insights. In conclusion, acquiring a thorough comprehension and incorporation of many aspects would enable a more knowledgeable and customized strategy to improve the chances of a healthy life and successful childbirth, particularly for women experiencing repeated and imminent pregnancy loss.

Conflict of interest

The author declares no conflict of interest.

Author details

Hisham Arab
Maternal and Fetal Health Program at Dr. Arab Medical Center, Jeddah, Saudi Arabia

*Address all correspondence to: arab123@gmail.com

References

[1] Kolatorova L, Vitku J, Suchopar J, Hill M, Parizek A. Progesterone: A steroid with wide range of effects in physiology as well as human medicine. International Journal of Molecular Sciences. 2022;**23**:(14):79-89

[2] Henderson VW. Progesterone and human cognition. Climacteric. 2018;**21**:333-340

[3] Bulletti C, Bulletti FM, Sciorio R, Guido M. Progesterone: The key factor of the beginning of life. International Journal of Molecular Sciences. 2022;**23**:14-38

[4] Taraborrelli S. Physiology, production and action of progesterone. Acta Obstetricia et Gynecologica Scandinavica. 2015;**94**:8-16

[5] Shah NM, Lai PF, Imami N, Johnson MR. Progesterone-related immune modulation of pregnancy and labor. Frontiers in Endocrinology. 2019;**10**

[6] Raghupathy R, Szekeres-Bartho J. Progesterone: A unique hormone with immunomodulatory roles in pregnancy. International Journal of Molecular Sciences. 2022;**23**

[7] Piette PCM. The pharmacodynamics and safety of progesterone. Best Practice and Research: Clinical Obstetrics and Gynaecology. 2020;**69**:13-29

[8] Mesiano S. Progesterone – Historical perspective. Journal of Steroid Biochemistry and Molecular Biology. 2022;**223**

[9] Micks E, Raglan GB, Schulkin J. Bridging progestogens in pregnancy and pregnancy prevention. Endocrine Connections. 2015;**4**(4):R81-R92

[10] Schindler AE, Campagnoli C, Druckmann R, Huber J, Pasqualini JR, Schweppe KW, et al. Classification and pharmacology of progestins. Maturitas. 2003;**46**(Suppl. 1):7

[11] Mitchell VE, Welling LLM. Not all Progestins are created equally: Considering unique Progestins individually in Psychobehavioral research. Adaptive Human Behavior and Physiology. 2020;**6**(3):381-412

[12] García-Sáenz M, Ibarra-Salce R, Pozos-Varela FJ, Mena-Ureta TS, Flores-Villagómez S, Santana-Mata M, et al. Understanding Progestins: From basics to clinical applicability. Journal of Clinical Medicine. 2023;**12**

[13] Sitruk-Ware R. Pharmacological profile of progestins. In: Maturitas. 2004. pp. 277-283

[14] Graham JD, Clarke CL. Physiological action of progesterone in target tissues* [Internet]. 1997. Available from: https://academic.oup.com/edrv/article/18/4/502/2530774

[15] Selcer KW, Leavitt' WW. Progesterone down-regulation of nuclear estrogen receptor: A fundamental mechanism in birds and mammals. General and Comparative Endocrinology. 1988;**12**(3):443-452

[16] Guerra JA, López-Muñoz F, Álamo C. Progestins in combined contraceptives. Journal of Experimental and Clinical Medicine(Taiwan). 2013;**5**:51-55

[17] Fedotcheva TA, Fedotcheva NI, Shimanovsky NL. Progesterone as an anti-inflammatory drug and immunomodulator: New aspects in hormonal regulation of the inflammation. Biomolecules. 2022;**12**(9):1299

[18] Louw-du Toit R, Storbeck KH, Cartwright M, Cabral A, Africander D. Progestins used in endocrine therapy and the implications for the biosynthesis and metabolism of endogenous steroid hormones. Molecular and Cellular Endocrinology. 2017;**441**:31-45

[19] Piette P. The history of natural progesterone, the never-ending story. Climacteric. 2018;**21**:308-314

[20] Griesinger G, Blockeel C, Kahler E, Pexman-Fieth C, Olofsson JI, Driessen S, et al. Dydrogesterone as an oral alternative to vaginal progesterone for IVF luteal phase support: A systematic review and individual participant data meta-analysis. PLoS ONE. 2020;**15**

[21] Colombo D, Ferraboschi P, Prestileo P, Toma L. A comparative molecular modeling study of dydrogesterone with other progestational agents through theoretical calculations and nuclear magnetic resonance spectroscopy. Journal of Steroid Biochemistry and Molecular Biology. 2006;**98**(1):56-62

[22] Katalinic A, Shulman LP, Strauss JF, Garcia-Velasco JA, van den Anker JN. A critical appraisal of safety data on dydrogesterone for the support of early pregnancy: A scoping review and meta-analysis. Reprod Biomed Online. 2022;**45**(2):365-373. DOI: 10.1016/j

[23] Rižner TL, Brožič P, Doucette C, Turek-Etienne T, Müller-Vieira U, Sonneveld E, et al. Selectivity and potency of the retroprogesterone dydrogesterone in vitro. Steroids. 2011;**76**(6):607-615

[24] Griesinger G, Tournaye H, Macklon N, Petraglia F, Arck P, Blockeel C, et al. Dydrogesterone: Pharmacological profile and mechanism of action as luteal phase support in assisted reproduction. Reproductive BioMedicine Online. 2019;**38**:249-259

[25] Schindler AE. Progestational effects of dydrogesterone in vitro, in vivo and on the human endometrium. Maturitas. 2009;**65**(Suppl. 1)

[26] Queisser-Luft A. Dydrogesterone use during pregnancy: Overview of birth defects reported since 1977. Early Human Development. 2009;**85**(6):375-377

[27] Podzolkova N, Tatarchuk T, Doshchanova A, Eshimbetova G, Pexman-Fieth C. Dydrogesterone treatment for menstrual-cycle regularization in routine clinical practice: A multicenter observational study. Gynecological Endocrinology. 2016;**32**(3):246-249

[28] Omar MH, Mashita MK, Lim PS, Jamil MA. Dydrogesterone in threatened abortion: Pregnancy outcome. Journal of Steroid Biochemistry and Molecular Biology. 2005;**97**(5):421-425

[29] El-Zibdeh MY, Yousef LT. Dydrogesterone support in threatened miscarriage. Maturitas. 2009;**65**(Suppl. 1)

[30] Pandian RU. Dydrogesterone in threatened miscarriage: A Malaysian experience. Maturitas. 2009;**65**(Suppl. 1)

[31] Carp H. A systematic review of dydrogesterone for the treatment of recurrent miscarriage. Gynecological Endocrinology. 2015;**31**:422-430

[32] Lee HJ, Park TC, Kim JH, Norwitz E, Lee B. The influence of oral dydrogesterone and vaginal progesterone on threatened abortion: A systematic review and meta-analysis. BioMed Research International. 2017;**2017**

[33] Haas DM, Hathaway TJ, Ramsey PS. Progestogen for preventing miscarriage

in women with recurrent miscarriage of unclear etiology. Cochrane Database of Systematic Reviews. 2018;**2018**

[34] Kale AR, Kale AA, Yelikar K. A comparative, randomized control trial in patients of per vaginal bleeding comparing efficacy of oral dydrogesterone versus vaginal progesterone in successful pregnancy outcome for patients with recurrent pregnancy loss. Journal of Obstetrics and Gynecology of India. 2021;**71**(6):591-595

[35] Zhao H, He W, Yang Z. A pairwise and network meta-analysis comparing the efficacy and safety of progestogens in threatened abortion. International Journal of Gynecology & Obstetrics. 2022;**156**:383-393

[36] Tetruashvili N, Domar A, Bashiri A. Prevention of pregnancy loss: Combining progestogen treatment and psychological support. Journal of Clinical Medicine. 2023;**12**

[37] Jamila N, Muhammad S, Wajiha A. The role of dydrogesterone in the medical management of 100 cases of dysfunctional uterine bleeding (DUB) above 35 years of age. Journal of Postgraduate Medical Institute [Internet]. 2011;**17**(2). Available from: https://jpmi.org.pk/index.php/jpmi/article/view/824

[38] Panay N, Pritsch M, Alt J. Cyclical dydrogesterone in secondary amenorrhea: Results of a double-blind, placebo-controlled, randomized study. Gynecological Endocrinology. 2007;**23**(11):611-618

[39] Karakus S, Kiran G, Ciralik H. Efficacy of micronised vaginal progesterone versus oral dydrogestrone in the treatment of irregular dysfunctional uterine bleeding: A pilot randomised controlled trial. Australian and New Zealand Journal of Obstetrics and Gynaecology. 2009;**49**(6):685-688

[40] Zaman T. Severity of bleeding is a predictor of quality of life in women with heavy menstrual bleeding under dydrogesterone treatment in a prospective, multicentre, observational study. Gazzetta Medica Italiana Archivio per le Scienze Mediche. 2015;**174**(9):391-398

[41] Trivedi N, Chauhan N, Vaidya V. Effectiveness and safety of dydrogesterone in regularization of menstrual cycle: A post-marketing study. Gynecological Endocrinology. 2016;**32**(8):667-671

[42] Solovyeva AV, Chegus LA. Abnormal uterine bleeding in women of reproductive age and premenopause. Akusherstvo i Ginekologiya (Russian Federation). 2020;**2020**(8):29-38

[43] Wang L, Guan HY, Xia HX, Chen XY, Zhang W. Dydrogesterone treatment for menstrual-cycle regularization in abnormal uterine bleeding - Ovulation dysfunction patients. World Journal of Clinical Cases. 2020;**8**(15):3259-3266

[44] Cagnacci A, Arangino S, Baldassari F, Alessandrini C, Landi S, Volpe A. A comparison of the central effects of different progestins used in hormone replacement therapy. Maturitas. 2004;**48**(4):456-462

[45] Drakopoulos P, Roelens C, De Vos M, Mackens S, Racca AL, Tournaye H, et al. The future of luteal phase support in ART and the role of Dydrogesterone. Frontiers in Reproductive Health. 2020;**2**

[46] Vidal A, Dhakal C, Werth N, Weiss JM, Lehnick D, Kohl Schwartz AS. Supplementary dydrogesterone is beneficial as luteal phase support in artificial frozen-thawed embryo

transfer cycles compared to micronized progesterone alone. Front Endocrinol (Lausanne). 2023;**14**

[47] Rashidi BH, Ghazizadeh M, Tehrani Nejad ES, Bagheri M, Gorginzadeh M. Oral dydrogesterone for luteal support in frozen-thawed embryo transfer artificial cycles: A pilot randomized controlled trial. Asian Pacific Journal of Reproduction. 2016;**5**(6):490-494

[48] Saharkhiz N, Zamaniyan M, Salehpour S, Zadehmodarres S, Hoseini S, Cheraghi L, et al. A comparative study of dydrogesterone and micronized progesterone for luteal phase support during in vitro fertilization (IVF) cycles. Gynecological Endocrinology. 2016;**32**(3):213-217

[49] Johnston WIH. Dydrogesterone and endometriosis. British Journal of Obstetrics and Gynaecology. 1916;**83**

[50] Schweppe KW. The place of dydrogesterone in the treatment of endometriosis and adenomyosis. Maturitas. 2009;**65**(Suppl. 1)

[51] Sukhikh GT, Adamyan LV, Dubrovina SO, Baranov II, Bezhenar VF, Kozachenko AV, et al. Prolonged cyclical and continuous regimens of dydrogesterone are effective for reducing chronic pelvic pain in women with endometriosis: Results of the ORCHIDEA study. Fertility and Sterility. 2021;**116**(6):1568-1577

[52] Peng C, Huang Y, Zhou Y. Dydrogesterone in the treatment of endometriosis: Evidence mapping and meta-analysis. Archives of Gynecology and Obstetrics. 2021;**304**(1):231-252

[53] Dubrovina SO, Berlim YD, Bezhenar VF, Gimbut VS, Baranov II. Pharmacological management of endometriosis-related pain: The expert opinion. Journal of SAFOG. 2020;**12**:415-420

[54] Liang B, Wu L, Xu H, Cheung CW, Fung WY, Wong SW, et al. Efficacy, safety and recurrence of new progestins and selective progesterone receptor modulator for the treatment of endometriosis: A comparison study in mice. Reproductive Biology and Endocrinology. 2018;**16**(1)

[55] Tagreed H, Mohanad M, Hayder F. Comparison of the efficacy and safety between dienogest and dydrogesterone in treatment of endometriosis: Prospective study. International Journal of Science and Research (IJSR) [Internet]. 2018;**7**(3):1704-1707. Available from: https://www.ijsr.net/archive/v7i3/ART20179838.pdf

[56] Huvinen E, Holopainen E, Heikinheimo O. Norethisterone and its acetate - What's so special about them? BMJ Sexual and Reproductive Health. 2021;**47**:102-109

[57] Bińkowska M. Menopausal hormone therapy and venous thromboembolism. Przeglad Menopauzalny. 2014;**13**(5):267-272

[58] Hellgren M, Conard J, Norris L, Kluft C. Cardiovascular risk markers during treatment with estradiol and trimegestone or dydrogesterone. Maturitas. 2009;**62**(3):287-293

[59] Ott J, Egarter C, Aguilera A. Dydrogesterone after 60 years: A glance at the safety profile. Gynecological Endocrinology. 2022;**38**:279-287

[60] Mattioli F, Garbero C, Gosmar M, Manfredi V, Carrozzino R, Martelli A, et al. DNA fragmentation, DNA repair and apoptosis induced in primary rat hepatocytes by dienogest, dydrogesterone and

1,4,6-androstatriene-17β-ol-3- one acetate. Mutation Research, Genetic Toxicology and Environmental Mutagenesis. 2004;**564**(1):21-29

[61] Tournaye H, Sukhikh GT, Kahler E, Griesinger G. A phase III randomized controlled trial comparing the efficacy, safety and tolerability of oral dydrogesterone versus micronized vaginal progesterone for luteal support in in vitro fertilization. Human Reproduction. 2017;**32**(5):1019-1027

[62] Yang DZ, Griesinger G, Wang W, Gong F, Liang X, Zhang H, et al. A phase III randomized controlled trial of oral dydrogesterone versus intravaginal progesterone gel for luteal phase support in in vitro fertilization (lotus II): Results from the Chinese mainland subpopulation. Gynecological Endocrinology. 2020;**36**(2):175-183

[63] Griesinger G, Blockeel C, Sukhikh GT, Patki A, Dhorepatil B, Yang DZ, et al. Oral dydrogesterone versus intravaginal micronized progesterone gel for luteal phase support in IVF: A randomized clinical trial. Human Reproduction. 2018;**33**(12):2212-2221

[64] Roux C, Kolta S, Chappard C, Morieux C, Dougados M, De Vernejoul MC. Bone effects of dydrogesterone in ovariectomized rats: A biologic, histomorphometric, and densitometric study. Bone. 1996;**19**

[65] Karami M, Mousavi SH, Rafiee M, Heidari R, Shahrokhi SZ. Biochemical and molecular biomarkers: Unraveling their role in gestational diabetes mellitus. Diabetology and Metabolic Syndrome. 2023;**15**

[66] Pergialiotis V, Bellos I, Hatziagelaki E, Antsaklis A, Loutradis D, Daskalakis G. Progestogens for the prevention of preterm birth and risk of developing gestational diabetes mellitus: A meta-analysis. American Journal of Obstetrics and Gynecology. 2019;**221**:429-436.e5

[67] Areeruk W, Phupong V. A randomized, double blinded, placebo controlled trial of oral dydrogesterone supplementation in the management of preterm labor. Scientific Reports. 2016;**6**

Section 3

The Clinical Application of Progesterone

Chapter 4

Progesterone: An Essential Diagnostic Resource in Veterinary Medicine

Nicolae Tiberiu Constantin, Florin Petrişor Posastiuc and Crina Raluca Andrei

Abstract

Progesterone (P4), a steroid hormone, is widely recognized for its vital function in maintaining pregnancy across various animal species. Its functions extend beyond pregnancy management, encompassing the determination of pregnancy, optimal reproductive timing, anticipation of parturition, scheduling of elective cesarean sections, and identification of conditions like growth hormone disorders, insulin-dependent diabetes, and infertility. Its versatility extends to involvement in bone marrow trophication, stress response assessment, and neuroprotection following traumatic brain injuries or fetal hypoxia. Although the aforementioned are mostly directed toward females, it is important to note that progesterone is also used clinically in males. Monitoring blood progesterone levels in animals is essential in both healthy and pathological states, as emphasized in this chapter.

Keywords: progesterone, endocrinology, diagnosis, small animals, large animals

1. Introduction

Despite nearly a century following its discovery by a group of researchers at the University of Rochester, there are still aspects of progesterone's role in the animals that make it in their bodies that remain to be understood. Undoubtedly, the absence of it would result in the absence of offspring, since it plays a crucial role in female cyclicity, preparing the uterus for gestation and ensuring its maintenance. It is classified as a progestogen, which is a kind of steroid hormone and is considered the most significant hormone in this category. In general, its functions are comparable in domestic animals, encompassing both reproductive and mammary gland aspects, as well as metabolic processes, since it is recognized as a neurosteroid.

Progesterone (P4) is produced by the corpus luteum, which forms following the release of the dominant follicle. Following that, several components including both large and tiny thecal cells, fibroblasts, and vascular elements will form a genuine endocrine gland that is accountable for producing progesterone and other compounds, depending on the specific species.

Alternatively, depending on the species, the placenta, which is the link between the mother and fetus, can sustain pregnancy by releasing several hormones, including the mentioned hormone.

Due to the wide range of reproductive and non-reproductive scenarios in which progesterone plays a role, it is crucial to provide a clear description of the specific instances in which this hormone might be utilized for diagnostic reasons. The objective of this chapter is to provide doctors with a realistic technique to assist them in assessing progesterone levels.

2. Progesterone's diagnostic reach in domestic carnivores

For domestic carnivores, prompt assessment of progesterone (P4) levels is essential for diagnosing conditions and making clinical decisions [1]. This includes the use of serum or plasma P4 measurements as diagnostic aids in various reproductive disorders such as pyometra, pseudopregnancy, ovarian remnant syndrome, hypoluteinism, ovarian cysts, or any form of disturbed estrus cycle such as silent estrus, split heat, or even delayed puberty/primary or secondary anestrus.

Additionally, the applications of P4 measurements extend to feline pregnancy diagnosis and pregnancy monitoring in both dogs and cats. Confirming P4 drops before parturition is essential for cesarean section (C-section) timing protocols [2]. Moreover, P4 is extensively used for ovulation determination and, consequently optimal breeding, the abrupt increase in P4 concentration during ovulation being a more reliable reference point when deciding on the "fertile window" when compared to the preovulatory peak LH concentration [3].

Progesterone's implications extend beyond the reproductive system, with research indicating its involvement in various areas such as neurodegenerative states and demyelination [4–6], as well as its association with conditions like dog hyperadrenocorticism [7] or adrenocortical tumors [8]. Additionally, progesterone has been linked to other metabolic influences, including its relationship with insulin activity and diabetes mellitus [9].

2.1 Estrus phase diagnosis and breeding management

In female dogs, the incipient luteinization process of granulosa cells prior to ovulation will translate into a noticeable rise in peripheral P4 concentrations. This particularity empowers us to use P4 as a diagnostic tool even before the start of the metestrus. Therefore, P4 levels under 1–2 ng/mL may be indicative of anestrus [10] or early to even persistent proestrus [11]. Further dynamics will prove a rapid elevation above 1 ng/mL during the preovulatory LH surge, with P4 plasma concentrations on the day of LH reaching 2.95 ± 1.2 ng/mL [12]. Subsequently, it undergoes further rapid escalation, either immediately or following a pause of 1–3 days, reaching levels of 10–25 ng/mL by day 10 of the cycle, typically occurring at or shortly after the end of estrus, post-ovulation [13].

In addition to clinical examination, vaginal cytology, vaginoscopy, LH assays, and ovarian ultrasound, P4 measurements were considered among the foremost methods utilized for monitoring the estrus cycle and diagnosing ovulation. This became essential for the utilization of cryopreserved material, enhancing assisted reproductive technology (ART) applications in small animal medicine.

However, P4 is able to significantly increase the diagnostic accuracy for ovulation prediction, and a standard value interval is hardly considered due to method and individual variability [14, 15]. Several groups compared different techniques for P4 analysis the ovulation range being cited as between 2.76 and 10 ng/mL [1, 10, 13–20].

In cats, P4 levels can also confirm ovulation. Breeding management recommendations suggest that serum P4 values exceeding 2 ng/mL at 1–2 weeks after mating indicate the presence of a luteal body [21]. When ovulation is pharmacologically induced, the success of this intervention can be checked by P4 measurements at 3–5 days distance [22].

2.2 Disturbed cycles

The abnormal cyclicity in the dog may refer to the failure of exhibiting estrus or to the unexpected duration of one of the phases including the interestrus interval. The first scenario may refer to primary or secondary anestrus. The age of puberty in female dogs' ranges from 6 to 14 months, with a diagnosis of primary anestrus potentially warranted if estrus has not occurred by 24 months of age [11]. The term secondary anestrus indicates that the patient has experienced at least one estrus cycle in the past but is currently unable to enter heat for several months (typically 12 months) [23]. Both conditions need to be distinguished from silent heat, missed heat, or drug-induced anestrus. Current recommendations suggest using P4 serum analysis for this purpose, with concentrations exceeding 2 ng/mL indicating that ovulation is imminent or has occurred within the last 2 months [24]. Moreover, recent approaches suggest that monthly P4 testing can be conducted to ascertain whether an unnoticed estrus has taken place in a supposedly non-cycling female dog [25]. In non-spayed felines, primary anestrus is usually ruled out similarly to the bitch taking into account any possible sexual development abnormality along with probable iatrogenic or environmental factors that may postpone puberty. On the other hand, for the secondary anestrus, P4 may actually reveal some important aspects such as lack of estrous due to a spontaneous ovulation not followed by pregnancy. In this case cyclicity will cease and P4 will remain high for 40–45 days [25].

Prolonged or persistent proestrus/estrus is another functional problem that may be detected in the bitch by the help of P4 monitorization. Even if the average duration for the proestrus period is still considered to be of 9 days, some females may exhibit signs of proestrus for up to 28 days until advancing to estrus [25]. Therefore, in suspected persistent estrus/proestrus cases, it is advisable to conduct vaginal cytology and progesterone testing [26]. Progressive cornification should match the increase in P4. On the contrary, if P4 reassessment proves no luteinization after 30 days of vaginal keratinization, that may indicate the evolution of an ovarian pathology with subsequent estrogenic stimulation and ovulation failure. Therefore, P4 may also guide the clinician in the diagnosis of follicular cysts or ovarian neoplasia.

Conversely, shorter interestrus intervals in bitches may be associated with two diverse situations: split heat or abbreviated metestrus/anestrus. The first stated condition will be clinically described as a female dog who exhibits estrus symptoms for a limited period of time without ovulating, followed by a silent interval and subsequent resumption of heat symptoms. Females experiencing a shortened metestrus and/or anestrus are those that enter heat again less than 4 months after an estrus period with confirmed ovulation. In terms of P4 testing the two situations may be differentiated, as during split-heat P4 does not rise above 2.0 ng/mL initially and this fact will be marked by the disappearance of estrus clinical signs and vaginal smear cornification [26]. The shortened luteal phase will be characterized by a consistent increase in P4 associated with a faster return to estrus.

Another rare cycle abnormality (1.2%) which usually evolves with a shorter interestrus interval is anovulation [27]. Primary cause of the latter, in dogs, is related to the failure of the ovary to deliver enough estrogen to elicit an LH surge [26] which will be equivalent to the insufficient mechanical stimulation during mating in the cat which will similarly produce insufficient LH release [28]. In both species the absence of ovulation can be highlighted through P4 serum determination, specific values being reported as under 2 ng/mL.

2.3 Detection of residual ovarian tissue

The ovarian remnant syndrome is a relatively frequent issue in veterinary practice, being reported as a complication in 17–43% ovariohysterectomy cases [29]. The detection of residual ovarian tissue can involve presumptive diagnosis through clinical observations, complemented by additional assessments such as vaginal cytology. Ultrasonography can also be employed as a diagnostic tool in this context. When considering slightly more invasive methods for diagnosing ovarian remnant syndrome, measuring concentrations of estradiol and P4, both before and after stimulation with gonadotropin-releasing hormone (GnRH) or human chorionic gonadotropin (hCG), as well as assessing luteinizing hormone (LH) or anti-Müllerian hormone (AMH) [30, 31], encompass the practical diagnostic possibilities. Lately a protocol combining P4 and AMH on the same serum sample proved to increase sensitivity for ovarian remnant syndrome diagnosis in dogs [29]. Even without stimulation, P4 alone can still be helpful in dogs, as progesterone concentrations may remain elevated for approximately 4 months out of a 12-month period, indicating the presence of functional luteal tissue. However, in queens, evaluating P4 may reliably detect ovarian tissue only if ovulation was induced.

2.4 Ovarian cysts

Functional ovarian cysts come in two types: follicular and luteal cysts. Furthermore, nonfollicular cysts may develop from the surface or subsurface epithelium and mesonephric tubules of the dog's ovary [32]. As primary diagnosis is achieved through clinical and ultrasonographical findings, definitory differential assessment of the cyst type relies on ovarian steroid hormone concentrations or histopathology. Follicular cysts typically induce a characteristic clinical buildup owing to their estrogenic influence. However, luteal cysts have the potential to extend the interestrus period, without any other clinical evidence. A diagnosis approach was proposed for these cases based on demonstrating the prolonged secretion of serum progesterone (>2 to 5 ng/mL) during 9- or 10-week period [33]. Moreover, a more invasive approach was also described based on the levels of oestradiol-17ß and progesterone concentration in the cystic fluid [34].

2.5 Progesterone dependent disorders of the reproductive tract

As a consequence of high progesterone levels associated with the normal luteal phase, various reproductive disorders may develop in both dogs and cats, including cystic endometrial hyperplasia, pyometra, pseudopregnancy, and mammary gland hyperplasia. For most of the stated pathological entities, P4 assessments may slightly increase diagnosis accuracy as it has the power to conclude on the estrus cycle phase, knowing the specificity of these disorders in relation to the metestrus. However, some particular pyometra cases including stump pyometra may benefit even more from P4 determination [35, 36]. Moreover, if medical treatment is attempted for pyometra, some authors consider serum P4 monitorization as being crucial in confirming the return to baseline levels after treatment initiation [37].

2.6 Pregnancy diagnosis and monitoring

P4 levels in female dogs remain elevated, whether they are pregnant or experiencing pseudopregnancy. Thus, by relying solely on progesterone levels, one cannot confirm pregnancy. However, monitoring progesterone is crucial in cases of complicated pregnancies, history of resorptions, abortions, or stillbirths. Additionally, determining the timing for parturition or C-sections in bitches can benefit from progesterone checks, as P4 levels typically fall 48–36 hours before parturition [24]. This differs for cats, as their progesterone concentrations decrease as parturition approaches but may not return to basal levels until after birth [38]. Consequently, progesterone levels cannot reliably predict parturition in cats. Conversely, P4 may provide late pregnancy diagnosis in felines. High P4 levels after 45 days of pregnancy, which coincides with the end of the possible pseudopregnancy, which may render a false positive, will prove placental progesterone production and therefore gestation [39]. However, this technique does not offer any information regarding the vitality of the embryo/fetus [40].

To effectively manage pregnancy, it is advisable to regularly do clinical examinations, ultrasounds, and P4 tests to detect any underlying conditions that might potentially impact the pregnancy. In cats, luteal insufficiency does not raise as many concerns as in dogs according to the different endocrine physiology. On the other hand, hypoluteoidism is considered among the potential explanations for pregnancy loss in dogs that undergo resorption, abortion, or premature whelping [24]. The consensus among most authors is that diagnosing hypoluteoidism in dogs involves ruling out all other potential causes of pregnancy loss, particularly infectious factors like *Brucella canis*, other opportunistic vaginal bacteria leading to uterine infection, Canine herpesvirus, or systemic diseases [41, 42]. If suspicion of hypoluteinism in a pregnant bitch persists, blood samples should be collected weekly, starting five to 7 days after the last breeding [43]. General recommendations state that a female is diagnosed with hypoluteinism and should be supplemented if P4 decreases below 5.0 ng/mL before the last week of pregnancy [43]. A detailed and more cautious approach was further proposed, considering that P4 levels ought to exceed 20.0 ng/mL from days 10 to 30, surpass 5.0 ng/mL from days 30 to 45, and remain above 1.5 ng/mL from days 45 to 58 [44]. According to the same authors, a sudden decline in progesterone by 10 to 15 ng/mL between days 20 and 35 suggests hypoluteoidism and signals a need for supplementation [44].

2.7 Parturition timing and elective C-section

When no data is available according to the LH peak or ovulation timing, together with ultrasonographical measurements, P4 assessments are important for parturition prediction or C-section scheduling. For a P4 level of 1 ng/mL, whelps are typically within 18–24 h; if P4 is below 1 ng/mL, early stages of whelp have either begun or will begin within 18 h [45].

C-section has been regarded as safe for both the bitch and the litter when progesterone levels decrease below 2 ng/mL [46]. Based on other studies, the threshold was set to 1.47 ng/mL [47]. Another approach stated that it is more important for the female to be within 48 hours of the spontaneous onset of parturition than to have a P4 level below 2 ng/mL for the safety of a programmed C-section [48]. Nevertheless, determining the stage of pregnancy often relies on P4 assessments meant to accurately pinpoint the day of the LH peak or ovulation, expecting normal parturition to take place 65 days ±1 or 63 days ±1 after the stated events [13]. Alternatively, serial vaginal cytology may be employed to ascertain the beginning of metestrus, considering that a scheduled C-section can be safely performed around 57 days after the start of the luteal phase [48].

2.8 Beyond reproduction

The impact of elevated progesterone levels in various metabolic disorders has been thoroughly examined, and its involvement in regulating glycemic levels has already been established [49]. Modern research highlighted that elevated P4 and P4-regulated growth hormone overexpression during metestrus or pregnancy pose a significant risk factor for the development of diabetes mellitus, particularly in older female dogs [9]. Therefore, P4 serum assessments were recommended as valuable tools in the initial screening of the entire diabetic female dog [9]. This approach allows the practitioner to understand the relationship between P4 stimulation and impaired insulin activity, thereby guiding him toward an appropriate intervention to improve the success of diabetes management.

Another application for P4 testing refers to advanced investigations related to occult hyperadrenocorticism, which was described as the situation in which history and clinical findings indicate hypercortisolism, but all stimulation tests fall into the accepted reference ranges [7]. The release of progesterone, along with 17-α-hydroxyprogesterone or other sex hormone or cortisol precursors, may inhibit pituitary adrenocorticotropic hormone secretion and lead to the degeneration of healthy adrenocortical tissue [50]. Analogously, serum P4 was proved to be useful for adrenocortical tumor diagnosis [8]. In such cases, progesterone-secreting adrenal tumors can cause specific hypercortisolism tests to yield negative results despite the presence of typical clinical signs and the tumor itself.

Progesterone has been associated with various neurodegenerative processes [4, 51]. However, investigations into distemper virus-infected dogs revealed no significance in either P4 serum levels or cerebrospinal fluid P4 [5]. Nevertheless, there was a significant decrease in cerebellum progesterone concentration [5], sparking future interest in this topic concerning various neurological conditions.

3. Progesterone's diagnostic reach in ruminants

3.1 Establishing the stage of sexual cycle in ruminants

In cattle, a decreasing trend of progesterone (P4) (in milk and in blood plasma) was observed before ovulation: in milk from <15 ng/mL (97.7 ± 17.8 hours before ovulation) to <5 ng/mL (79.7 ± 11.2 hours before ovulation), <2 ng/mL (70.7 ± 16.8 hours before ovulation) and in plasma from <4 ng/mL (90.5 ± 19.6 hours before ovulation) to <2 ng/mL (75.0 ± 12.2 hours before ovulation). Due to the wide range in the timing of progesterone concentrations dropping in relation to ovulation in different animals, it is recommended that progesterone monitoring is always accompanied by a transrectal ultrasound examination to determine the time of ovulation [52]. The onset of the luteal phase is represented by the increase in milk P4 concentration from <5 ng/mL to values > 5 ng/mL, and the luteal phase lasts as long as the P4 concentration is >5 ng/mL [53].

In goats, following the analysis of progesterone concentration in matched samples of feces and blood, a stunning similarity was observed between the patterns of progesterone variation throughout the sexual cycle. However, there are two differences: a slight delay in the evolution of progesterone in feces compared to plasma (1–2 days), and the values of progesterone concentration in feces are much higher compared to those in plasma (41.87 ± 2.16 ng/g vs. 0.36 ± 0.04 ng/mL in follicular phase and 241.31 ± 17 ng/g vs. 8.29 ± 0.56 ng/mL in the mid-luteal phase). This study is an experimental model, and the observed results can be used in the case of wild ruminants in which it is much easier to determine the stage of the sexual cycle by determining progesterone following the collection of feces than by blood samples [54]. In dairy goats, fecal progesterone concentration testing may offer an alternate technique for diagnosing early pregnancy and predicting estrus and parturition. Consequently, there was a noticeable decrease in the fecal progesterone levels 3 days before estrus was observed (until 396.9 ± 59.8 ng/g from 2957.6 ± 352.0 ng/g 5 days before estrus). The measurement of fecal progesterone levels 19–20 days after mating enables a precise diagnosis of pregnancy (1044.7 ng/g). The fecal progesterone profile appears to have increased gradually between weeks 7 and 14 of pregnancy, peaked between weeks 15 and 21, and then rapidly declined to start 5 to 6 days prepartum (5212.8 ± 463.6 ng/g), with a notable reduction occurring 1–2 days prepartum (3884.3 ± 576.0 ng/g). No significant correlation was observed between the concentration of progesterone from the feces and the number of kids born [55].

In general, buffalo ovulations are limited to P4 levels in milk and serum, which range from 0.1 to 2.9 ng/mL and 0.1 to 0.4 ng/mL, respectively. The mid-ovarian cycle P4 peak levels in milk and serum were found to vary between 6.7–17.8 ng/mL and 2.6–8.5 ng/mL, respectively. It was determined that in regularly monitored buffalo, a dramatic drop in milk P4 level to less than 2.9 ng/mL may serve as a reliable signal for when ovulation occurs [56].

3.2 Predicting pregnancy loss

In cattle, in order to determine if an early loss of pregnancy occurs, the plasma concentrations of progesterone and Pregnancy Specific Protein B (PSPB) can be measured on days 29–45 post-mating, the P4 variation being the decisive one. Thus, if the PSPB value is 0.6–1.1 ng/mL, but P4 < 2 ng/mL, the percentage of pregnancy loss in dairy cattle is higher than in the case of the same PSPB concentration, but with the level of P4 greater than 4 ng/mL [57].

3.3 Pregnancy diagnosis

In cattle, serum or milk progesterone can represent tools for early diagnosis of pregnancy, but with a precision that is not 100%. Samples are collected on days 21 and 24 post-artificial insemination, and if at least one sample has a low progesterone value, the female is non-pregnant. In other words, if the concentration of progesterone is high in both samples, the cow should be pregnant [58]. Pregnant animals have fecal progesterone concentrations of more than 50 ng/g on days 18–24 after artificial insemination or estrus, suggesting that feces can be used as an alternate for plasma and milk in measuring progesterone for the purpose of pregnancy diagnosis in heifers and cows [59].

According to a recent study, the approximately 7-day antepartum P4 and IGF-1 levels could be considered diagnostic markers for the following gestation [60].

In sheep, indication of pregnancy was established at a plasma progesterone level in ewes of ≥1.75 ng/mL [61]. Plasma progesterone concentration at day 18 post-mating is a reliable indication of fertilization success since it remains elevated in pregnant ewes while decreasing in ewes who did not conceive [62].

As in the case of ewes, it seems that an early pregnancy diagnosis can be made in buffaloes on the concentration of progesterone that will be higher in pregnant females than in non-pregnant ones on the 18th day after mating [63]. It seems that P4 concentrations in the serum and milk of pregnant buffalo varied from 2.0 to 8.5 ng/mL and 3.1 to 18.6 ng/mL, respectively, whereas the P4 levels in serum and milk of non-pregnant animals varied from 0.1 to 8.5 ng/mL and 0.1 to 19.9 ng/mL, respectively [56].

3.4 Diagnosis of luteal deficiency

In cattle, Intense metabolism, steroid hormone clearance from excessive milk production, heat stress, and other variables can all be implicated in low luteal activity, making it difficult or impossible to make an etiologic diagnosis [64]. Clinical diagnosis can be made using plasma or milk P4 concentrations in correlation with ovarian brightness (B)-mode ultrasonography or color-flow Doppler ultrasonography in order to monitories the luteal vascularization [65]. Up to day 40 of gestation, pregnant cows' plasma P4 concentrations, and luteal body blood flow have been found to positively correlate [66]. While an earlier (<7 days) or delayed (>11 days) onset of luteal activity post-artificial insemination has been linked to a lower pregnancy rate, there is a clear correlation between the rise in plasma P4 concentrations post-ovulation and the accomplishment of the pregnancy [63, 65].

3.5 Ovarian cysts

The symptoms of ovarian cysts in cattle typically include: anoestrus is most common, especially during the postpartum period; irregular estrus intervals or regular estrous cycles but lowered fertility; mucometra with normal estrous cycle lengths (if the follicular cysts persist); loss of tone of the female genital tract; behavioral changes (buller cow) which are characteristic of nymphomania (excessive mounting, standing, deeper tone) and erratic milk production. A rise in calving intervals brought on by the existence of such cysts causes the dairy industry to suffer large financial losses [67].

Progesterone concentrations in the peripheral circulation are generally higher in the case of luteal cysts compared to follicular cysts [68]. Limits of P4 concentration for a cyst to be considered luteal should be above 1 ng/mL (plasma) and up to 10 ng/mL (milk). A combination of diagnostic techniques, including transrectal palpation (flaccid uterus in the absence of a corpus luteum, thicker walls than a follicular cyst), transrectal ultrasonography (diameter of the cysts >20 mm), and plasma progesterone profiles, are needed to accurately diagnose the type of ovarian cysts [66, 69, 70].

In buffaloes, when the fluid from the ovarian structures was evaluated, it was observed a higher concentration of P4 in double ovulated (5.5 ng/mL) or normal (5.3 ng/mL) ovaries compared to the ovaries with the follicular cysts (4.7 ng/mL) [71].

However, these results are in contradiction with those of another study [72], in which the progesterone values in the fluid of follicular cysts are higher (49–62 ng/mL) compared to those in the fluid of normal follicles (0.02–27.46 ng/mL).

3.6 Progesterone as an indicator for caseous lymphadenitis

Due to the occurrence of infectious diseases like caseous lymphadenitis in sheep, which is caused by *Corynebacterium pseudotuberculosis*, small ruminant farmers face significant financial losses. This disease results in lower productivity, defined by weight loss, deficient milk and wool production, carcasses condemnation, and devaluation of leather, even though the majority of infected animals do not exhibit expressive clinical signs [73].

In a study that compared corpus luteum and progesterone concentrations on days 7 and 20 after mating, the luteal body's morphology and blood perfusion characteristics did not differ, suggesting that the natural infection caused by *C. pseudotuberculosis* did not result in macroscopic changes. On the other hand, progesterone concentrations on day 20 following mating showed a substantial difference between seropositive (11.69 ng/mL) and seronegative (4.34 ng/mL) ewes. It can be concluded that an infection with *C. pseudotuberculosis* may result in enhanced levels of progesterone in the serum, associated with an elevated specific antibody production [74].

4. Progesterone's use as a diagnostic tool in horses

4.1 Progesterone in correlation to breeding management

It is widely recognized that the mare is a long-day breeder species; therefore, we expect the reproduction season in the Northern Hemisphere to commence in the spring. So as to determine whether a mare has passed through the reproductive season, serial determination of P4 concentrations in plasma or saliva, which should be below 1 ng/mL, can be utilized [75].

Therefore, it was observed that during the reproductive season, there was a positive correlation ($r = 0.68$, $p < 0.05$) between the diameter of the follicles and the levels of P4 recorded from the follicular fluid. However, there was no correlation between the follicle diameter and the levels of P4 assessed from the peripheral venous blood [76].

Recent studies have found evidence suggesting that lower-than-ideal levels of postovulatory P4 may lead to higher rates of embryo death due to decreased endometrial activity in the early stages after ovulation [74, 75]. Therefore, administering progesterone after day 5 post-ovulation would enhance the chances of optimal embryo development [77] and proper chorionic girdle formation in mares [78], especially those that have experienced previous loss of conception product. However, this effect is not observed in young mares [79]. It is worth noting that progesterone receptors are not present in the endometrial epithelium of mares until day 20 post-ovulation [80]. Furthermore, the modification of progestin during the early stages of pregnancy results in enhanced composition of histotrophs in terms of the amino acids lysine and isoleucine [81], leading to a more balanced development of the embryo [78]. However, when there are low levels of P4 at the beginning of the luteal phase, it decreases the negative feedback from the hypothalamic-pituitary axis, which affects the maintenance of pregnancy through secondary luteal structures [82]. Nevertheless, it is important to acknowledge that supplementing with progestins, such as altrenogest, might result in changes to the mare's immune system and the development of masculine traits in the female fetus [83].

Progesterone is recognized as the hormone that prepares the uterus to receive the embryo and sustain pregnancy [84]. However, it is important to note that during the corpus luteum phase secretion; there is no increase in the blood flow to the endometrium. Therefore, the idea that a larger intake of progesterone in the uterus is not supported [85]. A recent study has found that a progesterone concentration of 6.49 ng/mL, 4 days after ovulation, is required to prime the uterus for receiving the blastocyst and ensuring successful pregnancy in embryo transfer technology [86]. According to the researchers, the vasculature of the corpus luteum, which was measured using Doppler ultrasonography, showed a positive correlation ($r = 0.63$, $p < 0.05$) with both the levels of progesterone and the day of embryo transfer [86].

In another study, it was found that mares diagnosed as pregnant at 14 days post-ovulation had a higher P4 level on day 5 post-ovulation (6.4 ± 3.0 ng/mL vs. 5.5 ± 3.3 ng/mL, $p = 0.02$) than those not diagnosed at the same time [87]. Moreover, double- and triple-gestation mares monitored at the same time interval had significantly higher P4 concentrations than single-gestation mares (9.6 ± 4.9 ng/mL vs. 5.8 ± 2.2 ng/mL, respectively; $p = 0.01$) [87].

4.2 Disturbed cycles

Despite the fact that the extension of the luteal phase is associated with uterine pathologies, in the case of mares, this phenomenon might occur under circumstances that are not yet fully understood. Approximately 10% of mares can ovulate during diestrus [88]. This phenomenon is characterized by secondary ovulation occurring more than 3 days after the initial ovulation during the follicular phase. If this secondary ovulation occurs beyond the 9th day following the primary ovulation, the luteal phase will be prolonged due to the lack of receptors for prostaglandin $F_{2\alpha}$ in the secondary formed luteal body [89]. Furthermore, the serum concentrations of P4 will be lower than normal levels [88].

4.3 Progesterone-dependent disorders of pregnancy

The maintenance of gestation in mammals is primarily attributed to P4. In mares, gestation is sustained in the initial phase by progesterone secreted by the primary corpus luteum and supplementary corpus luteum (P4 > 4 ng/mL) [90]. However, after day 175 of gestation [91], the level of this hormone drops below 1 ng/mL [84]. When the concentrations of P4 on days 5–7 after ovulation are within the range of >2.5 ng/mL and ≥ 4 ng/mL, they are classified as "suboptimal endogenous P4 concentrations" [87]. After this period, the intricate nature of hormones creates a new challenge in sustaining pregnancy in the mare. Cholesterol from the mother is transported to the fetus and serves as a precursor for pregnenolone (P5) [92]. The enzymes 3β-HSD and 5α-reductase, found in the fetal trophoblast and endometrium, convert P5 into P4 and 5α-dihydroprogesterone (5αDHP) [93]. During the later stages of pregnancy, there is a little rise in the amount of P4 hormone [94]. An immunoenzymatic analysis can indicate potential fetal disorders such as placentitis [95]. Therefore, for acute diseases that resolve within 7 days, P4 concentrations decline quickly. However, for chronic disorders that last for more than 8 days, values tend to increase [96]. Traditionally, the monitoring of these values is done using immunoassay. However, there is a problem with cross-reactivity with other progestins, ranging from 2 to 50%. Therefore, in recent years, liquid chromatography in tandem with mass spectrometry (LC-MS/MS) has been chosen as an alternative. This method can distinguish between P4 and 5αDHP in a single analysis and provide accurate quantitative measurements of these substances. In recent research, the authors found a significant association ($r = 0.753$, $p < 0.001$) between low P4 levels (< 6.07 ng/mL) at 14 days of gestation and a high amount of uterine edema during estrus. However, this correlation did not have a detrimental effect on the survivability of the embryos [97, 98].

Furthermore, it is worth noting that primary luteal failure can occur in this species, albeit it is an uncommon occurrence [99]. This phenomenon has been extensively described in the literature, as referenced by sources [94, 95]. Nevertheless, it remains uncertain whether the embryo perishes as a consequence of basic luteal failure or due to the inability of the mother to recognize the pregnancy [100]. In one of the mentioned cases, the levels of exogenous P4 were below 2 ng/mL from days 15 to 72. However, the pregnancy was successfully carried out after the administration of progestogen [100].

4.4 Postpartum progesterone-dependent disorders

Another research found that progesterone receptors in the endometrial glands and stroma of mares are more intense and frequent during the luteal phase compared to the follicular phase. However, no association with the endometritis was discovered [101]. This finding contradicts the outcomes of another group of researchers who reported that endometrial fibrosis significantly reduces the expression of P4 and estradiol receptors [102].

5. Progesterone's use as a diagnostic tool in pigs

5.1 Specific progesterone characteristics throughout the estrus cycle and gestation

When monitoring progesterone levels in sows, it is important to consider that the levels of P4 in blood drawn from the caudal vena cava are greater than those collected from the jugular vein [103]. Furthermore, the concentration of P4 is greater in the oviductal region compared to the bloodstream, indicating the undisputed function of this hormone in the release of spermatozoa from the oviductal region [104].

One specific characteristic of pig reproduction that is similar to the wild boar is the seasonal subfertility that happens between August and October in the Northern Hemisphere as a result of heat stress [102, 103]. Therefore, this subfertility leads to the production of small litter size, higher rates of abortion, delayed onset of sexual maturity, decreased rates of successful conception, and a longer interval between weaning to estrous [105]. New research on post-pubertal gilts revealed that higher temperature stress results in the development of smaller luteal bodies. However, these smaller luteal bodies have the ability to produce a greater amount of P4 per unit of luteal tissue [106]. Nevertheless, it is important to consider the influence of nutrition on the secretion of P4 and the subsequent survival of the embryo, particularly in the initial days after ovulation [107]. This effect is likely related to the regulation of the orexin system by P4 [108]. Therefore, subjecting pregnant sows to a period of 45 days of starvation during the first trimester of gestation led to 25% of the sows maintaining their pregnancy [109].

The proper operation of the corpus luteum requires a substantial and crucial intake of lipid-rich substances and IGF-1, which are essential for the production of P4. During the initial stages of pregnancy, namely after ovulation, the ovaries produce less progesterone (2 ng/mL after 6 hours) [104] because to its breakdown in the liver. Following that, there is a rapid surge in the period from day 10 to day 13 of gestation [107]. To further corroborate the statement, the following values serve as indicators:

- During the estrous cycle, the levels of a certain hormone called ng/mL fluctuate. On days 2–4, the average level is 7.2 ± 0.97 ng/mL. On days 10–12, the average level increases to 16.44 ± 2.18 ng/mL. On days 14–16, the average level drops to 1.03 ± 0.19 ng/mL. Finally, on days 18–20, the average level further decreases to 0.91 ± 0.18 ng/mL [109].

- During gestation, the levels of ng/mL also vary. On days 14–16, the average level is 21.24 ± 3.05 ng/mL. On days 30–32, the average level increases to 23.45 ± 3.39 ng/mL [110]. From days 30 to 105, the average level remains relatively stable, ranging from 18 to 25 ng/mL [109].

5.2 Lactation through the lens of progesterone

Effective control of parturition is crucial for the future well-being of newborn piglets. Specifically, in the case of pigs, pregnant females exhibit nest-building behavior when there is a fall in P4 levels and an increase in prolactin values before farrowing [111]. Furthermore, when females have a lack of or restricted access to various resources for constructing their nest, they will exhibit elevated P4 levels [112].

Recent research has found that there are positive connections between the quality or amount of colostrum and other factors influenced by the sow, which can ultimately result in the death of newborn piglets. Based on research, P4 levels were deemed to exceed the limitations at the beginning of farrowing when they were greater than 6 ng/mL and greater than 4.9 ng/mL at the end of the farrowing [113]. The authors found that 50% of the subjects had abnormal P4 values at both time points mentioned. They concluded that piglets born to sows with P4 values greater than 4.9 ng/mL at the end of parturition were more likely to develop neonatal diarrhea on the first day of life. The odds ratio was 3.71, with a confidence interval of 1.04–13.23 and a p-value of 0.04. This increased risk was attributed to low immunological levels.

Furthermore, elevated levels of progesterone during the initial 48 hours after farrowing might result in the birth of underdeveloped piglets, disrupt milk production and indicate that those sows had a big litter [114]. Contrarily, a little amount of P4 before farrowing results in an increase in the production of colostrum without any impact on its quality [115].

6. Conclusion

This chapter describes in as practical a way as possible the need to assess progesterone levels, often in combination with other hormones or medical procedures. Given the myriad practical applications in which it can be used, it is not wrong to use the term as a marker for certain physiological, but especially pathological, conditions. This capital is far from being considered complete, but we hope it will be exploited to the fullest until new studies improve the present work.

DOI: http://dx.doi.org/10.5772/intechopen.1005670

Acknowledgements

We are grateful to our colleagues and students from the Faculty of Veterinary Medicine at the University of Agronomical Sciences and Veterinary Medicine of Bucharest. We owe them who we are now as professionals.

Conflict of interest

The authors declare no conflict of interest.

Thanks

Deepest thanks to our mentors, families and faithful friends.

Author details

Nicolae Tiberiu Constantin*, Florin Petrişor Posastiuc and Crina Raluca Andrei
Faculty of Veterinary Medicine - University of Agronomic Sciences and Veterinary Medicine of Bucharest, Romania

*Address all correspondence to: tiberiu.constantin@fmvb.usamv.ro

References

[1] Fontbonne A, Maenhoudt C, Thoumire S, et al. Evaluation of surface plasmon field-enhanced fluorescence spectroscopy for rapid measurement of progesterone concentration in bitches. American Journal of Veterinary Research. 2021;**82**(5):417-424. DOI: 10.2460/ajvr.82.5.417

[2] De Cramer KGM, Nöthling JO. The precision of predicting the time of onset of parturition in the bitch using the level of progesterone in plasma during the preparturient period. Theriogenology. 2018;**107**:211-218. DOI: 10.1016/j.theriogenology.2017.11.018

[3] de Gier J, Kooistra HS, Djajadiningrat-Laanen SC, Dieleman SJ, Okkens AC. Temporal relations between plasma concentrations of luteinizing hormone, follicle-stimulating hormone, estradiol-17β, progesterone, prolactin, and α-melanocyte-stimulating hormone during the follicular, ovulatory, and early luteal phase in the bitch. Theriogenology. 2006;**65**(7):1346-1359. DOI: 10.1016/j.theriogenology.2005.08.010

[4] González SL, Labombarda F, Deniselle MCG, Guennoun R, Schumacher M, De Nicola AF. Progesterone up-regulates neuronal brain-derived neurotrophic factor expression in the injured spinal cord. Neuroscience. 2004;**125**(3):605-614. DOI: 10.1016/j.neuroscience.2004.02.024

[5] Yarim GF, Karahan S, Yarim M. Cerebellum progesterone concentration decreased in canine distemper virus infection. Research in Veterinary Science. 2007;**82**(2):173-180. DOI: 10.1016/j.rvsc.2006.05.008

[6] Lerouet D, Marchand-Leroux C, Besson VC. Neuropharmacology in traumatic brain injury: From preclinical to clinical neuroprotection? Fundamental & Clinical Pharmacology. 2021;**35**(3):524-538. DOI: 10.1111/fcp.12656

[7] Behrend EN, Kooistra HS, Nelson R, Reusch CE, Scott-Moncrieff JC. Diagnosis of spontaneous canine Hyperadrenocorticism: 2012 ACVIM consensus statement (small animal). Journal of Veterinary Internal Medicine. 2013;**27**(6):1292-1304. DOI: 10.1111/jvim.12192

[8] Farges A, Crawford D, da Silva CA, Ramsey I. Hyperprogesteronism associated with adrenocortical tumours in two dogs. Veterinary Record Case Reports. 2024;**12**(e794):1-9. DOI: 10.1002/vrc2.794

[9] Pöppl ÁG, Lopes JLX, Nogueira TB, da Silva DI, dos Santos MB. Progesterone-related diabetes mellitus in the bitch: Current knowledge, the role of Pyometra, and relevance in practice. Animals. 2024;**14**(6):890. DOI: 10.3390/ani14060890

[10] Hollinshead F, Hanlon D. Normal progesterone profiles during estrus in the bitch: A prospective analysis of 1420 estrous cycles. Theriogenology. 2019;**125**:37-42. DOI: 10.1016/j.theriogenology.2018.10.018

[11] Risvanli A, Ocal H, Kalkan C. Abnormalities in the sexual cycle of bitches. In: Canine Medicine - Recent Topics and Advanced Research. London, UK, London, UK: InTech; 2016. DOI: 10.5772/64648

[12] Guérin C, Maurel MC, Launais M, Delétang F, Badinand F. Use of an immunoenzymatic assay to detect the

luteinizing hormone peak in bitches. Journal of Reproduction and Fertility. Supplement. 1997;**51**:277-281

[13] Concannon PW. Reproductive cycles of the domestic bitch. Animal Reproduction Science. 2011;**124**(3-4):200-210. DOI: 10.1016/j.anireprosci.2010.08.028

[14] Jensen SØ, Öberg J, Alm H, Holst BS. Validation of a dry-slide immunoassay for progesterone analysis in canine plasma in a clinical setting. Veterinary Clinical Pathology. 2022;**51**(4):524-532. DOI: 10.1111/vcp.13140

[15] Kunanusont N, Punyadarsaniya D, Ruenphet S. Accuracy and precision guidelines for optimal breeding time in bitches using in-house progesterone measurement compared with chemiluminescent microparticle immunoassay. Veterinary World. 2021;**14**(3):585-588. DOI: 10.14202/vetworld.2021.585-588

[16] Zuercher J, Boes KM, Balogh O, Helms AB, Cecere JT. Comparison of a point-of-care Analyzer with a Chemiluminescent immunoassay for serum progesterone measurement in breeding Management of the Bitch. Frontiers in Veterinary Science. 2021;**8**:1-9. DOI: 10.3389/fvets.2021.660923

[17] Kustritz MVR. Managing the reproductive cycle in the bitch. The Veterinary Clinics of North America. Small Animal Practice. 2012;**42**(3):423-437. DOI: 10.1016/j.cvsm.2012.01.012

[18] Groppetti D, Aralla M, Bronzo V, Bosi G, Pecile A, Arrighi S. Periovulatory time in the bitch: What's new to know? Animal Reproduction Science. 2015;**152**:108-116. DOI: 10.1016/j.anireprosci.2014.11.008

[19] Milani C, Boscato EL, Gabai G, et al. Analytical and clinical performance of a fluorescence enzyme immunoassay for progesterone and determination of ovulation day in bitches. Journal of Veterinary Diagnostic Investigation. 2022;**34**(6):977-982. DOI: 10.1177/10406387221125466

[20] Johnston SD. Clinical approach to infertility in bitches with primary Anestrus. The Veterinary Clinics of North America. Small Animal Practice. 1991;**21**(3):421-425. DOI: 10.1016/S0195-5616(91)50051-6

[21] Johnson AK. Breeding and cattery management. In: Feline Reproduction. Boston: CABI; 2022. pp. 41-46. DOI: 10.1079/9781789247107.0004

[22] Goericke-Pesch S, Packeiser E-M. Reproductive Management in Catteries: Optimising health and wellbeing through veterinarian-breeder collaboration. Journal of Feline Medicine and Surgery. 2022;**24**(9):881-904. DOI: 10.1177/1098612X221118760

[23] Gobello C, Castex G, Corrada Y. Use of cabergoline to treat primary and secondary anestrus in dogs. Journal of the American Veterinary Medical Association. 2002;**220**(11):1653-1654. DOI: 10.2460/javma.2002.220.1653

[24] Johnston SD, Root Kustritz MV, Schultz OP. In: Company WS, editor. Canine and Feline Theriogenology. 1st ed. Philadelphia: Saunders; 2001

[25] Wilborn RR, Maxwell HS. Clinical approaches to infertility in the bitch. The Veterinary Clinics of North America. Small Animal Practice. 2012;**42**(3):457-468. DOI: 10.1016/j.cvsm.2012.01.016

[26] Meyers-Wallen VN. Unusual and abnormal canine estrous cycles. Theriogenology. 2007;**68**(9):1205-1210. DOI: 10.1016/j.theriogenology.2007.08.019

[27] Arbeiter K. Anovulatory ovarian cycles in dogs. Journal of Reproduction and Fertility. Supplement. 1993;**47**:453-456

[28] Fontbonne A, Niewiadomska Z. Causes of infertility in the queen. In: Feline Reproduction. Boston: CABI; 2022. pp. 47-55. DOI: 10.1079/9781789247107.0005

[29] Place NJ, Cheraskin J-L, Hansen BS. Evaluation of combined assessments of serum anti-Müllerian hormone and progesterone concentrations for the diagnosis of ovarian remnant syndrome in dogs. Journal of the American Veterinary Medical Association. 2019;**254**(9):1067-1072. DOI: 10.2460/javma.254.9.1067

[30] Axnér E, Holst BS. Concentrations of anti-Müllerian hormone in the domestic cat. Relation with spay or neuter status and serum estradiol. Theriogenology. 2015;**83**(5):817-821. DOI: 10.1016/j.theriogenology.2014.11.016

[31] Mullikin K, Byron M, Chen J, Cheong SH, Gartley C, de Amorim MD. Ovarian remnant syndrome in small animals: Case series. Clinical Theriogenology. 2022;**14**(4):370-377. DOI: 10.58292/ct.v14i4.9174

[32] Pires MA, Payan-Carreira R. Cystic structures in the canine ovary: A prevalence survey. In: EVSSAR, editor. 17th EVSSAR Conference-Reproduction and Pediatrics in Dogs, Cats and Exotic Carnivores. Wroclaw: EVSSAR; 2017. p. 179

[33] Fontbonne A. Infertility in bitches and queens: recent advances Infertilidade na cadela e gata: atualidades. Revista Brasileira de Reprodução Animal. 2011;**35**(2):202-209. Available from: www.cbra.org.br

[34] Knauf Y, Bostedt H, Failing K, Knauf S, Wehrend A. Gross pathology and endocrinology of ovarian cysts in bitches. Reproduction in Domestic Animals. 2014;**49**(3):463-468. DOI: 10.1111/rda.12311

[35] Ehrhardt C, Odunayo A, Pascutti K, Carvajal J, Ham K, Harris AN. Stump pyometra in a spayed female dog secondary to tamoxifen. Veterinary Medicine and Science. 2023;**9**(1):47-52. DOI: 10.1002/vms3.1041

[36] Xavier RGC, Santana CH, de Castro YG, et al. Canine Pyometra: A short review of current advances. Animals. 2023;**13**(21):3310. DOI: 10.3390/ani13213310

[37] Johnson A. Diagnosis and medical treatment of pyometra in the queen. Clinical Theriogenology. 2022;**14**(3):151-154. DOI: 10.58292/ct.v14i3.9165

[38] Holst BS. Feline breeding and pregnancy management: What is normal and when to intervene. Journal of Feline Medicine and Surgery. 2022;**24**(3):221-231. DOI: 10.1177/1098612X221079708

[39] Roos J, Fontbonne A. Pregnancy diagnosis and management. In: Feline Reproduction. Boston: CABI; 2022. pp. 56-73. DOI: 10.1079/9781789247107.0006

[40] Levy X, England GCW. Pregnancy diagnosis, normal pregnancy and parturition in the queen. In: BSAVA Manual of Canine and Feline Reproduction and Neonatology. London: British Small Animal Veterinary Association; 2010. pp. 98-105. DOI: 10.22233/9781905319541.11

[41] Graham EM, Taylor DJ. Bacterial reproductive pathogens of cats and dogs. The Veterinary Clinics of North America. Small Animal Practice. 2012;**42**(3):561-582. DOI: 10.1016/j.cvsm.2012.01.013

[42] Verstegen J, Dhaliwal G, Verstegen-Onclin K. Canine and feline pregnancy loss due to viral and non-infectious causes: A review. Theriogenology. 2008;**70**(3):304-319. DOI: 10.1016/j.theriogenology.2008.05.035

[43] Root Kustritz MV. Use of supplemental progesterone in Management of Canine Pregnancy. In: Concannon PW, England G, Verstegen J III, Linde Forsberg C, editors. Recent Advances in Small Animal Reproduction. Ithaca: International Veterinary Information Service; 2001

[44] Becher A, Wehrend A, Goericke-Pesch S. Luteale Insuffizienz bei der Hündin – Symptome, Diagnose, Folgen und Therapie. Tierärztliche Prax Ausgabe K Kleintiere/Heimtiere. 2010;**38**(06):389-396. DOI: 10.1055/s-0038-1622870

[45] Dolf G, Gaillard C, Russenberger J, Moseley L, Schelling C. Factors contributing to the decision to perform a cesarean section in Labrador retrievers. BMC Veterinary Research. 2018;**14**(1):1-9. DOI: 10.1186/s12917-018-1381-8

[46] Smith FO. Challenges in small animal parturition—Timing elective and emergency cesarian sections. Theriogenology. 2007;**68**(3):348-353. DOI: 10.1016/j.theriogenology.2007.04.041

[47] Nöthling JO, Joonè CJ, Hegarty E, Schooley EK, De Cramer KGM. Use of a point-of-care progesterone assay to predict onset of parturition in the bitch. Frontiers in Veterinary Science. 2022;**9**:1-6. DOI: 10.3389/fvets.2022.914659

[48] De Cramer KGM, Nöthling JO. Towards scheduled pre-parturient caesarean sections in bitches. Reproduction in Domestic Animals. 2020;**55**(S2):38-48. DOI: 10.1111/rda.13669

[49] Eigenmann JE, Eigenmann RY, Rijnberk A, van der Gaag I, Zapf J, Froesch ER. Progesterone-controlled growth hormone overproduction and naturally occurring canine diabetes and acromegaly. Acta Endocrinologica. 1983;**104**(2):167-176. DOI: 10.1530/acta.0.1040167

[50] Syme HM, Scott-Moncrieff JC, Treadwell NG, et al. Hyperadrenocorticism associated with excessive sex hormone production by an adrenocortical tumor in two dogs. Journal of the American Veterinary Medical Association. 2001;**219**(12):1725-1728. DOI: 10.2460/javma.2001.219.1725

[51] Schumacher M, Guennoun R, Robert F, et al. Local synthesis and dual actions of progesterone in the nervous system: Neuroprotection and myelination. Growth Hormone & IGF Research. 2004;**14**:18-33. DOI: 10.1016/j.ghir.2004.03.007

[52] Roelofs JB, Van Eerdenburg FJCM, Hazeleger W, Soede NM, Kemp B. Relationship between progesterone concentrations in milk and blood and time of ovulation in dairy cattle. Animal Reproduction Science. 2006;**91**(3-4):337-343. DOI: 10.1016/j.anireprosci.2005.04.015

[53] Bruinjé TC, Colazo MG, Ribeiro ES, Gobikrushanth M, Ambrose DJ. Using in-line milk progesterone data to characterize parameters of luteal activity and their association with fertility in Holstein cows. Journal of Dairy Science. 2019;**102**(1):780-798. DOI: 10.3168/jds.2018-14654

[54] Hirata S, Mori Y. Monitoring reproductive status by Fecal progesterone

analysis in ruminants. The Journal of Veterinary Medical Science. 1995;**57**(5):845-850. DOI: 10.1292/jvms.57.845

[55] Jack AMM, Chang CC, Peh HC, Chan JPW. Fecal progesterone analysis for monitoring reproductive status in dairy goats. Turkish Journal of Veterinary & Animal Sciences. 2012;**36**(5):566-572. DOI: 10.3906/vet-1105-1

[56] Osman K, El-Regalaty H, Fekry A, Farghaly H, Aboul-Ela H. Use of milk progesterone assay for monitoring ovulation, ovarian cycles and pregnancy in buffalo. Journal of Animal and Poultry Production. 2010;**1**(5):163-174. DOI: 10.21608/jappmu.2010.86199

[57] Gábor G, Kastelic J, Abonyi-Tóth Z, Gábor P, Endrődi T, Balogh O. Pregnancy loss in dairy cattle: Relationship of ultrasound, blood pregnancy-specific protein B, progesterone and production variables. Reproduction in Domestic Animals. 2016;**51**(4):467-473. DOI: 10.1111/rda.12703

[58] Bekele N, Addis M, Abdela N, Ahmed WM. Pregnancy diagnosis in cattle for fertility management: A review. Global Veterinary. 2016;**16**(4):355-364. DOI: 10.5829/idosi.gv.2016.16.04.103136

[59] Isobe N, Akita M, Nakao T, Yamashiro H, Kubota H. Pregnancy diagnosis based on the fecal progesterone concentration in beef and dairy heifers and beef cows. Animal Reproduction Science. 2005;**90**(3-4):211-218. DOI: 10.1016/j.anireprosci.2005.02.004

[60] Constantin NT, Bercea-Strugariu CM, Bîrțoiu D, et al. Predicting pregnancy outcome in dairy cows: The role of IGF-1 and progesterone. Animals. 2023;**13**(10):1579. DOI: 10.3390/ani13101579

[61] Codreanu I, Codreanu M. Study regarding hormonal and biochemical profiles in pregnant and lactating ewes treated with bromocriptine. Scientific Works C Series; LVII(3):54-57

[62] Ganaie BA, Khan MZ, Islam R, Makhdoomi DM, Qureshi S, Wani GM. Evaluation of different techniques for pregnancy diagnosis in sheep. Small Ruminant Research. 2009;**85**(2-3):135-141. DOI: 10.1016/j.smallrumres.2009.09.003

[63] Codognoto VM, Souza FF, Salgado LC, et al. Can blood progesterone concentration identify non-pregnant buffaloes to support oestrous resynchronization. Reproduction in Domestic Animals. 2022;**57**(6):673-677

[64] Kornmatitsuk B, Chantaraprateep P, Kornmatitsuk S, Kindahl H. Different types of postpartum luteal activity affected by the exposure of heat stress and subsequent reproductive performance in Holstein lactating cows. Reproduction in Domestic Animals. 2008;**43**(5):515-519. DOI: 10.1111/j.1439-0531.2007.00945.x

[65] López-Gatius F, Garcia-Ispierto I. Clinical overview of luteal deficiency in dairy cattle. Animals. 2022;**12**(15):1-7. DOI: 10.3390/ani12151871

[66] Beindorff N, Nagai K, Shirasuna K, et al. Vascular changes in the corpus luteum during early pregnancy in the cow. The Journal of Reproduction and Development. 2010;**56**(2):263-270. DOI: 10.1262/jrd.09-150K

[67] Jeengar K, Chaudhary V, Kumar A, Raiya S, Gaur M, Purohit GN. Ovarian cysts in dairy cows: Old and new concepts for definition. Diagnosis and Therapy. 2014;**11**(2):63-73

[68] Ochea M, Pascal M, Şonea A, Bîrţoiu AI. The effect of epidural administration of FSH in bovine superovulation protocol. Animal Science. 2015;**58**:217-220

[69] Spencer TE, Forde N, Lonergan P. The role of progesterone and conceptus-derived factors in uterine biology during early pregnancy in ruminants1. Journal of Dairy Science. 2016;**99**(7):5941-5950. DOI: 10.3168/jds.2015-10070

[70] Turner ZB, Lima FS, Conley AJ, et al. Cystic ovarian disease in dairy cattle: Diagnostic accuracy when using B-mode and color Doppler ultrasound. Journal of Dairy Science. 2023;**106**(5):3411-3420. DOI: 10.3168/jds.2022-22498

[71] Zeitoun MM. Effect of physiological status of buffalo ovaries on progesterone and biochemical constituents in follicular fluids. In: Proceedings of the 26th Annual Meeting of the Brazilian Embryo Technology Society (SBTE). Alexandria: SBTE; 2012

[72] Khan FA, Nabi SU, Pande M, Das GK, Sarkar M. Bilateral follicular cysts in a water buffalo. Tropical Animal Health and Production. 2011;**43**(3):539-541. DOI: 10.1007/s11250-010-9738-4

[73] Pépin M, Paton MW. Caseous lymphadenitis in sheep and goats. In: Lefevre PC, Blancou J, Chermette R, Uilenberg G, editors. Infectious and Parasitic Disease of Livestock. 1st ed. Paris: Lavoisier; 2010. 1153 p

[74] Costa JO, Barral TD, Portela RD, et al. Correlation between the natural infection by Corynebacterium pseudotuberculosis in goats and serum progesterone levels and corpus luteum development. Domestic Animal Endocrinology. 2022;**78**:106677. DOI: 10.1016/j.domaniend.2021.106677

[75] Goudet G, Douet C, Pianos A, et al. Saliva and plasma steroidome in mare during reproductive stages: A GC-MS/MS study. Frontiers in Animal Science. 2022;**3**(October):1-18. DOI: 10.3389/fanim.2022.1055179

[76] Satué K, Fazio E, Ferlazzo A, Medica P. Intrafollicular and systemic serotonin, oestradiol and progesterone concentrations in cycling mares. Reproduction in Domestic Animals. 2019;**54**(10):1411-1418. DOI: 10.1111/rda.13545

[77] Willmann C, Budik S, Walter I, Aurich C. Influences of treatment of early pregnant mares with the progestin altrenogest on embryonic development and gene expression in the endometrium and conceptus. Theriogenology. 2011;**76**(1):61-73. DOI: 10.1016/j.theriogenology.2011.01.018

[78] Okada CTC, Kaps M, Reichart U, et al. Low plasma progesterone concentration during the early luteal phase delays endometrial development and the beginning of placentation in mares. Animal Reproduction Science. 2022;**247**:1-12. DOI: 10.1016/j.anireprosci.2022.107149

[79] Willmann C, Schuler G, Hoffmann B, Parvizi N, Aurich C. Effects of age and altrenogest treatment on conceptus development and secretion of LH, progesterone and eCG in early-pregnant mares. Theriogenology. 2011;**75**(3):421-428. DOI: 10.1016/j.theriogenology.2010.05.009

[80] Wilsher S, Gower S, Allen WRT. Immunohistochemical localisation of progesterone and oestrogen receptors at the placental interface in mares during early pregnancy. Animal Reproduction Science. 2011;**129**(3-4):200-208. DOI: 10.1016/j.anireprosci.2011.11.004

[81] Beyer T, Rink BE, Scarlet D, Walter I, Kunert S, Aurich C. Early luteal phase progestin concentration influences endometrial function in pregnant mares. Theriogenology. 2019;**125**:236-241. DOI: 10.1016/j.theriogenology.2018.11.018

[82] Okada CTC, Kaps M, Quesada JP, Gautier C, Aurich J, Aurich C. Diestrous ovulations in pregnant mares as a response to low early postovulatory progestogen concentration. Animals. 2020;**10**(12):1-9. DOI: 10.3390/ani10122249

[83] Fedorka CE, Troedsson MHT. The use of progestins in equine medicine: A review. Equine Veterinary Education. 2021;**33**(9):494-504. DOI: 10.1111/eve.13332

[84] Wynn MAA, Esteller-Vico A, Legacki EL, et al. A comparison of progesterone assays for determination of peripheral pregnane concentrations in the late pregnant mare. Theriogenology. 2018;**106**:127-133. DOI: 10.1016/j.theriogenology.2017.10.002

[85] Ginther OJ, Beg MA. Dynamics of circulating progesterone concentrations before and during luteolysis: A comparison between cattle and horses. Biology of Reproduction. 2012;**86**(6):1-12. DOI: 10.1095/biolreprod.112.099820

[86] Sales FABM, Vasconcelos Azevedo M, Matos Souza N, et al. Correlations of corpus luteum blood flow with fertility and progesterone in embryo recipient mares. Tropical Animal Health and Production. 22 Apr 2021;**53**(2):280. DOI: 10.1007/s11250-021-02583-9

[87] Hollinshead FK, Mehegan MK, Gunn A, Nett T, Bruemmer JE, Hanlon DW. The correlation of endogenous progesterone concentration in Diestrus on early pregnancy rate in thoroughbred mares. Journal of Equine Veterinary Science. 2022;**118**:104127. DOI: 10.1016/j.jevs.2022.104127

[88] Von Hippel FA. The reproductive cycle. Tinbergen's Leg Behav Sixty Years Landmark Stickleback Paper. 2010;**8**(December):23-39. DOI: 10.1163/ej.9789004170292.i-540.7

[89] Ginther OJ. Prolonged luteal activity in mares - a semantic quagmire. Equine Veterinary Journal. 1990;**22**(3):152-156. DOI: 10.1111/j.2042-3306.1990.tb04235.x

[90] Shideler RK, Squires EL, Voss JL, Eikenberry DJ, Pickett BW. Progestagen therapy of ovariectomized pregnant mares. Journal of Reproduction and Fertility. 1982;**32**(459-464):16

[91] Popova M. Breeding age of mares from the Haflinger breed, duration of gestational length and the influence of some Paratype factors on it. Scientific Papers. Series D. Animal Science. 2020;**LXIII**(1):263-270

[92] Chavatte P, Holtan D, Ousey JC, Rossdale PD. Biosynthesis and possible biological roles of progestagens during equine pregnancy and in the newborn foal. Equine Veterinary Journal. Supplement. 1997;**24**(24):89-95. DOI: 10.1111/j.2042-3306.1997.tb05084.x

[93] Han X, Rossdale PD, Ousey J, et al. Localisation of 15-hydroxy prostaglandin dehydrogenase (PGDH) and steroidogenic enzymes in the equine placenta. Equine Veterinary Journal. 1995;**27**(5):334-339. DOI: 10.1111/j.2042-3306.1995.tb04067.x

[94] Conley AJ. Review of the reproductive endocrinology of the pregnant and parturient mare. Theriogenology. 2016;**86**(1):355-365. DOI: 10.1016/j.theriogenology.2016.04.049

[95] Ousey JC, Houghton E, Grainger L, Rossdale PD, Fowden AL. Progestagen profiles during the last trimester of gestation in thoroughbred mares with normal or compromised pregnancies. Theriogenology. 2005;**63**(7):1844-1856. DOI: 10.1016/j.theriogenology.2004.08.010

[96] Morris S, Kelleman AA, | Stawicki RJ, et al. Transrectal ultrasonography and plasma progestin profiles identifies feto-placental compromise in mares with experimentally induced placentitis. Theriogenology. 2007;**67**(4):681-691. DOI: 10.1016/j.theriogenology.2006.05.021

[97] Grabowska A, Kozdrowski R. Relationship between estrus endometrial edema and progesterone production in pregnant mares two weeks after ovulation. BMC Veterinary Research. 2022;**18**(1):1-8. DOI: 10.1186/s12917-022-03512-0

[98] Allen WR. Luteal deficiency and embryo mortality in the mare. Reproduction in Domestic Animals. 2001;**36**(3-4):121-131. DOI: 10.1046/j.1439-0531.2001.d01-43.x

[99] Vanderwall DK, Squires EL, Brinsko SP, McCue PM. Diagnosis and management of abnormal embryonic development characterized by formation of an embryonic vesicle without an embryo in mares. Journal of the American Veterinary Medical Association. 2000;**217**(1):58-63. DOI: 10.2460/javma.2000.217.58

[100] Canisso IF, Beltaire KA, Bedford-Guaus SJ. Premature luteal regression in a pregnant mare and subsequent pregnancy maintenance with the use of oral altrenogest. Equine Veterinary Journal. 2013;**45**(1):97-100. DOI: 10.1111/j.2042-3306.2012.00559.x

[101] Rojas D, Cabezas J, Ramírez G, Saravia F, Rodriguez-Alvarez L, Castro FO. Complimentary diagnostic tools for endometrosis in biopsies of mares with clinical subfertility. Acta Scientiae Veterinariae. 2020;**48**(1):1-9. DOI: 10.22456/1679-9216.98312

[102] Hoffmann C, Bazer FW, Klug J, Aupperle H, Ellenberger C, Schoon HA. Immunohistochemical and histochemical identification of proteins and carbohydrates in the equine endometrium. Expression patterns for mares suffering from endometrosis. Theriogenology. 2009;**71**(2):264-274. DOI: 10.1016/j.theriogenology.2008.07.008

[103] Virolainen JV, Love RJ, Tast A, Peltoniemi OAT. Plasma progesterone concentration depends on sampling site in pigs. Animal Reproduction Science. 2005;**86**(3-4):305-316. DOI: 10.1016/j.anireprosci.2004.07.004

[104] Mirihagalle S, Hughes JR, Miller DJ. Progesterone-induced sperm release from the oviduct sperm reservoir. Cells. 2022;**11**(10):1-13. DOI: 10.3390/cells11101622

[105] Bertoldo M, Holyoake PK, Evans G, Grupen CG. Follicular progesterone levels decrease during the period of seasonal infertility in sows. Reproduction in Domestic Animals. 2011;**46**(3):489-494. DOI: 10.1111/j.1439-0531.2010.01695.x

[106] Bidne KL, Romoser MR, Ross JW, Baumgard LH, Keating AF. Heat stress during the luteal phase decreases luteal size but does not affect circulating progesterone in gilts. Journal of Animal Science. 2019;**97**(10):4314-4322. DOI: 10.1093/jas/skz251

[107] Langendijk P, Peltoniemi O. How does nutrition influence luteal function and early embryo survival.

Bioscientifica Proceedings. 2019;**1**:145-158. DOI: 10.1530/biosciprocs.19.0015

[108] Dobrzyn K, Smolinska N, Kiezun M, et al. The in vitro effect of progesterone on the orexin system in porcine uterine tissues during early pregnancy. Acta Veterinaria Scandinavica. 2018;**60**(1): 1-14. DOI: 10.1186/s13028-018-0430-4

[109] Hard DL, Anderson LL. Maternal starvation and progesterone secretion, litter size, and growth in the pig. American Journal of Physiology-Endocrinology and Metabolism Gastrointestinal Physiology. 1979;**6**(3):273-278. DOI: 10.1152/ajpendo.1979.237.3.e273

[110] Skowronska A, Mlotkowska P, Eliszewski M, Nielsen S, Skowronski MT. Expression of aquaporin 1, 5 and 9 in the ovarian follicles of cycling and early pregnant pigs. Physiological Research. 2015;**64**(2):237-245. DOI: 10.33549/physiolres.932825

[111] Yun J, Swan KM, Farmer C, Oliviero C, Peltoniemi O, Valros A. Prepartum nest-building has an impact on postpartum nursing performance and maternal behaviour in early lactating sows. Applied Animal Behaviour Science. 2014;**160**(1):31-37. DOI: 10.1016/j.applanim.2014.08.011

[112] Yun J, Swan KM, Vienola K, et al. Nest-building in sows: Effects of farrowing housing on hormonal modulation of maternal characteristics. Applied Animal Behaviour Science. 2013;**148**(1-2):77-84. DOI: 10.1016/j.applanim.2013.07.010

[113] Hasan SMK, Junnikkala S, Valros A, Peltoniemi O, Oliviero C. Validation of brix refractometer to estimate colostrum immunoglobulin G content and composition in the sow. Animal. 2016;**10**(10):1728-1733. DOI: 10.1017/S1751731116000896

[114] De Passille AMB, Rushen J, Foxcroft GR, Schaefers A. Performance of Young Pigs: Relationships with Periparturient Progesterone, Prolactin, and Insulin of Sows'. Available from: https://academic.oup.com/jas/article-abstract/71/1/179/4632101

[115] Loisel F, Farmer C, van Hees H, Quesnel H. Relative prolactin-to-progesterone concentrations around farrowing influence colostrum yield in primiparous sows. Domestic Animal Endocrinology. 2015;**53**:35-41. DOI: 10.1016/j.domaniend.2015.04.005

Chapter 5

Use of Progesterone as a Strategy to Improve Reproductive Efficiency in Cattle

Samuel Rodrigues Bonamichi do Couto, Lara Nogueira Silenciato, Mariana dos Santos Dutra Okada, Otávia Reis e Silva, Joaquim Esquerdo Ferreira and Marco Roberto Bourg de Mello

Abstract

Progesterone (P4) is a key hormone in the reproductive physiology of cattle, playing a crucial role in regulating the estrous cycle and establishing and maintaining the pregnancy. In the context of reproductive efficiency, the use of P4 has been a strategy increasingly used on rural properties to anticipate puberty, increase pregnancy rates and reduce gestational loss. A common application is the administration of P4, often in the form of intravaginal devices or, more recently, with long-acting injectable progesterone. These methods help synchronize ovulation, allowing more precise management of reproductive programs, facilitating the use of artificial insemination, and contributing to genetic improvement. The synchronization of ovulation in beef and dairy cattle allows insemination at a pre-determined time without the need for estrus detection. These treatments increase the number of inseminated animals and, consequently, the number of pregnant animals. Overall, the strategic use of P4 in livestock management serves as a valuable tool for increasing reproductive efficiency, facilitating better control of reproductive cycles, and contributing to increased pregnancy rates and better overall reproductive performance in cattle herds.

Keywords: reproduction, cattle, hormone, progestin, conception rate

1. Introduction

In cattle, one of the factors causing infertility is related to the inadequate functioning of the corpus luteum (CL), which is characterized by a low peripheral concentration of progesterone. A deficiency in the secretion of this steroid hormone by the CL can contribute to the occurrence of embryonic and fetal losses, negatively impacting reproductive efficiency.

Progesterone is related to the maintenance of pregnancy and has a positive effect on the possibility of embryonic survival. In this context, strategies to increase the plasma concentration of progesterone would benefit embryonic development, improve pregnancy rates and reduce gestational loss.

As an attempt to improve the productive and reproductive indices of dairy and beef cattle, several studies have been carried out based on hormonal protocols for inducing puberty, synchronizing estrus and ovulation, promoting an increase in pregnancy rate and reducing gestational loss, with progesterone and progestins present among these studied hormones [1].

Common strategies implemented in cattle farming include (i) applications of human chorionic gonadotropin (hCG) or gonadotropin-releasing hormone (GnRH) to provide final support for follicular development and formation of an accessory corpus luteum [2]; (ii) exogenous P4 supplementation via slow-release intravaginal devices, orally, subcutaneously or even the use of long-acting injectable progesterone. All of these strategies aim to increase the concentrations of circulating P4 directly or indirectly, contributing beneficially to the elongation of the conceptus and the establishment of pregnancy in cattle, as already demonstrated in studies [3, 4].

2. Importance of progesterone in cattle

Substances capable of maintaining pregnancy and promoting the modification of the proliferative endometrium into a secretory one are classified as gestagens [5]. Among these substances, progesterone is of great relevance. Progesterone is a steroid hormone derived from cholesterol [6, 7], synthesized in the corpus luteum by small luteal cells and mainly by large luteal cells [8].

According to Binelli [9], P4 is related to the process of ovulation and the maintenance of pregnancy. It modulates follicular growth and exerts several functions in the growth of the endometrial and tubuloalveolar glands of the mammary gland. P4 acts in the regulation of gonadotropin secretion, in blocking the expression of estrus and ovulation by hypothalamic action; it also has an influence on the secretory activity of the oviduct and in the endometrial glands for the development of the zygote before its implantation and acts in the inhibition of contraction uterus and the maintenance of pregnancy [9–13].

Progesterone receptors are expressed during the luteal phase and are directly regulated by the concentration of P4 [14]. According to Wiltbank et al. [7], the concentration of P4 is regulated by the development of the CL after the pulsatile wave of luteinizing hormone (LH), more precisely by the number of granulosa cells that undergo the luteinization process, becoming large luteal cells, which begin to produce progesterone.

In cattle, plasma progesterone concentrations exhibit variation throughout the estrous cycle, with concentrations below 1 ng/ml during estrus and on the 10th day of the cycle, these concentrations vary between 2 and 3 ng/ml for zebu cows [15] and 16 ng/ml in taurine cows, such as the Holstein breed [16].

According to Bazer et al. [17], it is believed that P4 induces changes in gene expression and secretion and trophoblast formation, probably affecting the development of the conceptus. An increase in P4 concentration during metestrus and at the beginning of diestrus was related to the establishment of pregnancy after embryo transfer [18]. Other authors suggest that the concentration of P4 has an indirect effect on embryonic survival and development through the positive modulation of interferon-τ (IFN-τ) production, related to the recognition of pregnancy and inhibition of prostaglandin secretion and consequent luteolysis [4, 10].

Thus, females with reduced P4 concentrations at the beginning of diestrus could have an impaired pregnancy rate due to interference with fetal development and maternal recognition of pregnancy, with P4 being implicated in the process by stimulating the expression of some genes that favor embryo development, and the production of IFN-τ at the most appropriate time [9].

Although there is evidence that increasing P4 concentration has a positive effect on embryo development and fertility results, the results of studies that aimed to increase plasma concentrations of P4 are still inconclusive and conflicting [19].

Numerous anti-luteolytic strategies have been studied to enhance embryonic quality and reproductive efficiency in cattle. Among the strategies used are the formation of an accessory corpus luteum, through the application of hormones such as hCG or GnRH or even exogenous P4 supplementation via slow-release devices, orally, subcutaneously, or even the use of long-acting injectable progesterone [20–22].

3. Use of progesterone in inducing puberty in heifers

In the context of reproductive efficiency, age at first calving is directly related to the female's reproductive lifespan. By starting the heifer to reproduce earlier, the young female will have a greater production of calves throughout her productive life [23]. Therefore, the sexual precocity of females is a characteristic of great economic impact and has significant importance in reducing the generation interval, as the sooner the females can reproduce and become pregnant, the shorter the generation interval will be and the greater the genetic gain [24].

Aiming to improve productivity and reproductive efficiency, protocols with P4 supplementation were developed before timed artificial insemination (TAI) protocols to promote earlier puberty in heifers. The justification for this association is to increase the number of pubescent heifers at the beginning of the ovulation synchronization protocol and, consequently, maximize conception rates in TAI [25]. These protocols have used intravaginal devices [26], melengestrol acetate – MGA [27], and long-acting injectable P4 [25] as sources of progestin.

The anticipation of puberty and increased fertility of a herd directly reflect on profitability. Females younger than their first birth spend less time in the herd, leading to an increase in the number of calves born and, consequently, a greater economic return to the producer. However, achieving this goal is especially challenging in *Bos indicus* cattle because puberty generally occurs at older ages than in *Bos taurus*, ranging from 16 to 40 months. Possible causes of delay in reaching puberty are associated with genetic and environmental factors, including nutrition, disease, temperature, humidity and time of birth.

Breeding systems with heifers' first calving age at 24 months have higher productivity compared to those with first calving at 36–48 months of age. In induction protocols, progesterone in association with estrogen allows the induction of puberty in heifers, as P4 artificially simulates the functional state of the CL, allowing follicular growth, which results in greater estrogen production by the ovarian follicles and LH peak. Treatments with only progestins are capable of inducing puberty in heifers, although the result is influenced by the age, weight, body and follicular development of the heifers before treatment, highlighting that the exclusive use of P4 would be capable of inducing puberty only in those in which the negative estrogen feedback would have already started to decline [28].

The use of P4 as a pre-synchronization strategy is based on the fact that this hormone leads to a reduction in the number of estradiol receptors in the hypothalamus, interfering with the negative feedback caused by this hormone in GnRH secretion [29]. Furthermore, the use of P4 can increase receptors and their sensitivity to estrogen in the regions most sensitive (mediobasal hypothalamus) to the effect of estradiol on LH secretion [30].

Intravaginal progesterone devices that have already been used at least once have lower amounts of P4, and this results in a more efficient response in induction protocols, as they induce the formation of larger follicles, a higher estrus detection and conception rates, when compared to females treated with new devices [31]. High concentrations of progesterone are not beneficial for pre-pubertal heifers, as they can suppress LH pulsatility, thus impairing follicular development and ovulation, consequently affecting the results of puberty induction [32].

Anderson et al. [33] reported a positive effect of P4 (norgestomet) for 10 days on the induction of puberty, frequency of LH pulses and uterine weight of pre-pubertal heifers slaughtered 1 day before device removal. The authors observed anticipation of puberty (P4: 22 ± 9 d vs. control: 63 ± 12.5 d), increased uterine weight (P4: 222.3 ± 30 g vs. control: 72.7 ± 10.9 g), and increased number of LH pulses in heifers treated with P4. These authors concluded that treatment with progestins is effective in anticipating puberty and sexual maturity in cattle.

It has been demonstrated that progesterone is an efficient alternative for inducing puberty in cattle, aiming to facilitate management, reduce the generation interval and accelerate genetic gain. Vrisman et al. [34] monitored the luteal dynamics of Nellore heifers that were subjected or not to puberty induction with an intravaginal P4 device for 10 days, followed by the application of GnRH 48 hours after removing the device. In conclusion, the authors showed the importance of exposing pre-pubertal heifers to progesterone, as indicated by the higher percentage of CLs with normal function in the first estrous cycle compared to animals in the control group.

Satisfactory results of puberty induction and pregnancy were also reported by Lima et al. [25] by supplementing pre-pubertal Nellore heifers with long-acting injectable progesterone and, 10 days later, applying estradiol benzoate and prostaglandin. Twelve days after the end of the protocol, the animals were synchronized to observe heat and perform artificial insemination. The pregnancy rates reported by the authors were 46% for the group with puberty induction by P4 versus 38.3% for the control group.

Regarding the time between puberty induction and the beginning of the synchronization protocol to perform TAI, some studies indicate that an interval of more than 30 days between the beginning of induction and insemination provided a higher reproductive tract score and a higher pregnancy rate after TAI, compared to animals subjected to TAI a maximum of 30 days after induction [35].

It is important to highlight that in treatments to anticipate puberty, there are individual variations in the response to the administration of progesterone, and the effectiveness of P4 in anticipating puberty can be influenced by factors such as genetics, nutritional and environmental conditions.

In summary, the literature suggests that administering progesterone can effectively accelerate puberty in cattle, offering advantages in terms of reproductive and economic efficiency. Nonetheless, it is crucial to adopt an individualized approach and comprehend the factors that might impact the response to progesterone therapy.

4. Strategies for increasing progesterone after insemination

4.1 Exogenous progesterone supplementation

The current understanding of the role of progesterone during the early stage of pregnancy and in embryonic development has led to a series of studies on P4 supplementation after insemination, with a direct relationship between the ability to secrete P4 by the corpus luteum and embryonic growth, and the establishment of pregnancy [36]. This way, high concentrations of P4 during the initial phase of diestrus in cattle are fundamental, as they help with endometrial secretions, favoring embryonic development and the production of interferon-τ, related to the recognition of pregnancy and inhibition of prostaglandin secretion and luteolysis [10, 17, 36, 37].

The ability to produce interferon-τ in sufficient quantities depends on uterine stimuli, with P4 being involved in the process by stimulating the expression of some genes that favor embryonic development [9]. Therefore, females with low concentrations of P4 at the beginning of diestrus could have lower pregnancy rates due to interference in embryonic development and pregnancy recognition.

Exogenous P4 supplementation is an alternative to increase plasma progesterone concentrations. This supplementation can be carried out through the use of an intravaginal P4 device, administration of daily injectable doses of P4, administration of long-acting injectable P4, and supply of progestins in the diet, such as the use of melengestrol acetate [12, 22, 38, 39].

In a meta-analytic study, Wiltbank et al. [7] observed that P4 supplementation during diestrus, between days 3 and 7 of the estrous cycle, significantly increased the size of the conceptus on days 13 and 16 [4, 10]. Ababneh et al. [40] evaluated the effect of P4 supplementation (vaginal device) at different times of the estrous cycle of Holstein cows and observed a better conception rate between days 2 and 7 compared to cows treated between days 7 and 16. In another study, a better conception rate was observed with P4 supplementation (CIDR®) between days 5 and 19 compared to non-supplemented cows when evaluating the effects of post-insemination P4 administration in Holstein cows (control = 25%, CIDR = 56%) [41].

In a meta-analysis study carried out by Yan et al. [12] focusing on post-insemination progesterone supplementation in cattle, the authors observed that the strategy proved to be efficient when supplementation was carried out between days 3 and 7 after insemination, harmful when animals were supplemented before day 3 (for induce early luteolysis) and indifferent when performed after 7 days. These same authors also pointed out that supplementation is only efficient in herds in which the animals have compromised fertility (i.e., conception rate < 45%), resulting from ovulation deficiency or even insufficient concentrations of progesterone to sustain pregnancy in the initial phase.

The optimal timing for progesterone (P4) supplementation remains a subject of inquiry, as certain studies have reported neutral or even adverse outcomes. Parr et al. [42], when supplementing dairy cows with a P4 device between days 4 and 9 post-insemination, they observed a lower conception rate for treated animals. Possible explanations for this result involve a failure in CL development or even early luteolysis related to the previous increase in P4 exogenously. To prove these explanations, these same authors, in another study [43], showed that heifers with failed CL development, when supplemented with exogenous P4 from D4 to D10 (D0 = day of insemination), did not reverse these effects, demonstrating that P4 has a negative effect on the useful life of this CL, however, when supplemented from D4 to D7, there was a recovery of

CL area. These results may be directly related to LH pulsatility in this initial phase, since there is an inverse relationship between P4 concentration and LH pulse, where the primary developing CL depends on LH receptors in theca and granulosa cells, thus making it very vulnerable to hormonal variation [29].

In addition to the variation in LH pulsatility, it was demonstrated that P4 supplementation from D4 led to a decrease in the number of P4 receptors and an increase in CL oxytocin receptors on D5, but more studies are needed to investigate the effects of supplementation. of P4 on the development of CL [43].

Other forms of post-insemination P4 supplementation have already been tested, such as the use of MGA, a synthetic progestin formulated to be administered orally. Junior et al. [22] used MGA together with mineral salt, 2.28 g/day, starting 5 or 13 days after TAI, in 99 Nellore cows. The conception rate in the control group was 18% (n = 55), and in the group treated with MGA, the conception rate was 48.7% ($P < 0.05$). In the same study, the authors found no difference in pregnancy loss between 30 and 80 days.

Silva et al. [44] reported positive results when providing MGA to Nellore cows 13 to 18 days after TAI; however, when provided between days 5 and 10 post-TAI, the group treated with MGA showed a significant reduction in the pregnancy rate. These authors believe that this progestin in question has a different mode of action than the others, in which it does not favor the uterine environment during initial diestrus.

An alternative to increasing the concentration of P4 in the initial diestrus is the application of long-acting injectable P4 (P4LA). The aim of using this route of administration is to facilitate management, especially in beef herds, as it excludes a second management when compared to the use of intravaginal devices, which need to be removed after a few days [38]. P4LA at doses of 150 or 300 mg has been shown to increase circulating P4 concentrations for more than 3 days during the early luteal phase in beef cattle [3]. In summary, no differences were found between the use of intravaginal devices or the application of injectable P4LA for supplementation in early diestrus [12].

The use of injectable P4 has been studied for decades, as demonstrated by Johnson et al. [45], where the authors evaluated supplementation with 100 mg of P4LA on days 2, 3, 4, 5 and 9 after TAI, totaling 500 mg P4/animal, and found a higher pregnancy rate in treated animals compared to those from group control.

This strategy of supplementation with injectable P4LA has gained prominence in recent years. Pugliesi et al. [38], after several experiments evaluating the supplementation of injectable P4LA in beef cattle 4 days after TAI, demonstrated that this is an efficient strategy when there are animals with a deficient CL. For example, in animals that are in anestrus at the beginning of the TAI protocol (common in lactating beef cows raised on pasture), generating a 20% increase in the pregnancy rate. Likewise, Couto et al. [46], evaluating the supplementation of injectable P4LA on D5 in beef cattle (D0 = TAI), observed an increase in pregnancy rates and lower pregnancy loss in the treated group, highlighting the efficiency of administering P4 in early diestrus to improve herd fertility. Both studies suggest that supplementation at this stage improves the uterine environment and, consequently, the survival, elongation and implantation of the embryo, obtaining better results.

Furthermore, according to Couto et al. [47], the application of P4LA, 7 days after ovulation, was able to improve conception rates in animals with a reactive temperament, with increased cortisol levels, suggesting that supplementation is effective in animals that are subjected to some factor that could compromise basal progesterone levels, such as handling stress and low nutritional status.

According to Mann and Lamming [48], the increase in conception rates occurs only when P4 is supplemented in the first week after insemination and has no effect when exogenous P4 is supplemented in the second and third weeks after insemination.

In a study carried out with long-acting injectable P4, it was shown that a dose of 150 mg on the third day after TAI was a viable strategy to improve the conception rate; however, an anticipation of luteolysis was observed in some animals [3]. According to O'hara et al. [49], this same effect was observed in animals supplemented through an intravaginal device 3 days after TAI.

Martins et al. [50] investigated the impact of supplementing Nellore cows with long-acting injectable progesterone (P4LA) 3 days after timed artificial insemination (TAI). Their study evaluated the effect on early luteolysis and concluded that while P4 favors uterine receptivity, it can also reduce the longevity of the CL, making it difficult to establish pregnancy, since conceptus signaling cannot overcome the early luteolytic stimulus. Furthermore, early luteolysis is more related to the result of early exposure of the uterus to P4, which leads to the anticipation of the activation of the luteolytic cascade (production of PGF2alpha), than to the impairment of CL development due to the decrease in LH pulsatility. Additionally, these same authors [50] concluded that early luteolysis, due to the effect of P4 supplementation in animals that presented three follicular waves, was lower, suggesting that the number of follicular waves after AI plays a significant role in the fertility response to P4 supplementation, by regulating uterine function.

4.2 Induction of accessory corpus luteum

To counteract potential deficiencies in corpus luteum function, progesterone supplementation or the administration of luteotropic agents after ovulation is a viable approach [51]. According to Bech-Sabat et al. [52], cows normally produce a single CL after ovulation, but there are ways to induce the formation of an accessory corpus luteum to increase P4 concentrations. Administration of GnRH, GnRH agonists, or hCG at specific times after TAI can induce the formation of an accessory CL [53].

The use of these hormones and the consequent formation of accessory CL increases the plasma concentration of P4 and reduces the production of estradiol, producing a positive effect on embryonic development [54]. According to Besbaci et al. [55], studies on the subject have failed to provide a consensus on the benefits of such treatments since some report a beneficial effect of using GnRH or hCG in relation to pregnancy. In contrast, others do not show the same results [56].

Previous studies have shown that administration of GnRH, a GnRH agonist or hCG after TAI, in the presence of a dominant follicle in the first or second follicular waves, can induce the formation of accessory CL, increase P4 and reduce estrogen production [57]. According to Araújo et al. [58], ovulation of a first-wave follicle after TAI may alter follicular dynamics at the time of luteolysis, prolonging the time for luteolysis and allowing more time for embryo elongation.

Cows with an accessory corpus luteum were 0.32 times less likely to lose a pregnancy than cows with only one corpus luteum [39]. According to Lopez-Gatius et al. [59], cows that received GnRH on the day of TAI and 12 days later were 3.7 more likely to present accessory CL than cows that did not receive any dose. Beltran and Vasconcelos [53] observed that serum P4 concentrations increased from the 7th to the 12th day with GnRH injection applied on day 5 post-TAI about untreated animals.

Administration of GnRH, 5 days after TAI, in dairy cows increased P4 concentration on the 13th day after TAI; however, pregnancy rates were not different between the GnRH and control groups [60]. Ataman et al. [61] evaluated the use of GnRH (20 μg buserelin) 12 days after TAI and its effect on P4 concentration and pregnancy rate in dairy cows. Pregnant cows that received GnRH had higher P4 concentrations between days 18 and 21 compared to pregnant cows that received saline solution. Despite the difference observed in P4 concentrations between days 18 and 21, pregnancy rates between days 21 and 45 were not different.

In another study, Pinto et al. [62], evaluating induction of accessory corpus luteum and conception in embryo recipients, observed that 51% of treated animals had accessory corpora lutea while the control had 23.5% ($P = 0.04$). Additionally, the GnRH group demonstrated a conception rate of 38%, whereas the control group had 24% ($P < 0.05$).

In a meta-analytic study involving 52 articles on induction of accessory corpus luteum and the effect on pregnancy, it was observed that treatments with GnRH and hCG improve pregnancy in cows with low fertility (very low <30% and low 30.1 to 45%). On the other hand, the treatment of cows with high fertility (>60.1%) did not result in any benefit [55]. This study also reports that treatment with a medium or high dose (≥ 10 μg) of buserelin was associated with a higher conception rate than low doses of buserelin.

Stojanov et al. [63], evaluating the application of GnRH 5 days after insemination, observed an increase in the percentage of cows with more than two CLs on day 14 in the group treated with GnRH compared to the control group (82 vs. 0%). Furthermore, cows in the GnRH group that had accessory CL had higher P4 concentrations on day 14 (5.87 ± 2.04 ng/ml) compared to the control (4.21 ± 1.22 ng/ml) and the GnRH cows that did not present an accessory corpus luteum (only 1 CL on days 14–3.21 ± 1.12 ng/ml). On day 21, the conception rate was still higher in the GnRH group compared to control (65% vs. 48.3%, $p < 0.05$).

In a subsequent study, the effectiveness of GnRH and hCG administered 7 days post-insemination was investigated. Results revealed that 50% of animals treated with GnRH (lecerylin acetate) developed accessory corpus luteum, while in the hCG group, this proportion increased to 80%. Moreover, both the GnRH and hCG groups demonstrated significantly higher conception rates compared to the control group [64].

According to Stevenson et al. [57], there is a linear and positive relationship between the number of follicles ≥5 mm at the time of treatment (between 4 and 9 days post-AI) with GnRH or hCG and the number of CLs induced, with animals with 1 or 2 follicles ≥5 mm had fewer CLs induced than those with 4 or more follicles of the same size. In beef cows, the effect of hCG is similar to the effect in dairy cows, with this hormone capable of inducing ovulation when used 7 days after TAI. Therefore, it was observed that the number of accessory CLs was greater with hCG when compared to the use of saline (control group). Additionally, on day 33, the proportion of pregnant cows that had accessory CLs was higher in the hCG group than in the control group [56]. In another study evaluating the administration of buserelin (GnRH analog), an increase in the number of accessory corpora lutea was observed; however, this fact was not able to increase plasma concentrations of P4 and the conception rate [62].

In summary, the use of GnRH as an alternative to increase reproductive rates is well-studied, but the results are still controversial. The differences in results reported in the literature are consequences of many methodologies adopted, such as the moment of application and the GnRH analog used [47, 55, 63].

Studies aimed at evaluating the effect of the side formation of the accessory CL (contralateral or ipsilateral to the primary CL) on its maintenance during the first and second months of pregnancy have been developed. Accessory CL that was induced contralateral to the pregnancy CL tended to regress in 66% of pregnant cows around the 67th day of gestation. There were two different periods of regression of the contralateral CL in pregnant dairy cows: (I) close to the normal period of regression of a CL in non-pregnant cows (19 to 25 days of the cycle); (II) during the second month of pregnancy (30 to 60 days) [65].

Monteiro et al. [66] carried out a study to evaluate the time and serum concentrations of P4 associated with the regression of the contralateral accessory CL during the first and second months of pregnancy. The results showed that in pregnant cows, only the accessory CL contralateral to the pregnant CL underwent luteolysis. Functional luteolysis occurred quickly, with less than 24 hours for a drop in circulating P4 concentrations and between 48 and 96 hours for regression of luteal volume, both in the group that underwent early luteolysis (between 19 and 21 days) and in the group that underwent the process in the second month (between days 48 and 51). This speed and punctuality in the process suggest that the luteolytic mechanism is similar in both periods. Regarding the fact that there is no luteolysis of the CL ipsilateral to the pregnant CL, it is suggested that there is some protective mechanism for both during the second month of pregnancy. This mechanism may be related to the increase in uterine blood flow in the gravid horn.

It is known that the side of the accessory CL affects fertility, as multiparous cows have lower fertility than primiparous cows if the accessory CL is contralateral to the gravid CL. Likewise, the contralateral accessory CL is more likely to undergo early luteolysis (gestation less than 32 days) in multiparous cows than primiparous cows [65]. The regression of the accessory CL both in the early period (between days 19 and 23) and in the late period (>45 days) results in approximately 40% reduction in circulating P4 concentrations; therefore, the presence of an ipsilateral CL can be very more positive for fertility than that of a contralateral CL, especially if the regression of this accessory CL occurs during the early phase of pregnancy [66, 67].

In brief, the use of GnRH as an alternative to improve reproductive rates has been increasingly studied, but it still presents controversial and sometimes inconsistent results. The differences in results found in the literature are a consequence of the variety of methodologies used, mainly concerning the moment of application and the GnRH analog used.

5. Conclusion

The use of progesterone has been demonstrated to be an effective tool to optimize reproductive efficiency in cattle undergoing a timed artificial insemination program. The exogenous administration of this hormone makes it possible to induce puberty in heifers and control the females' estrous cycle, synchronizing them for artificial insemination at strategically chosen times. This not only makes herd management easier but also increases conception rates and reduces calving intervals, resulting in more efficient production. However, it is crucial to consider the appropriate dosage, timing of administration and specific herd conditions to ensure the success of the insemination program. In short, progesterone plays a fundamental role in optimizing reproductive efficiency in cattle, contributing to significant improvements in the productivity and profitability of animal production systems.

Conflict of interest

The authors declare no conflict of interest.

Author details

Samuel Rodrigues Bonamichi do Couto[1], Lara Nogueira Silenciato[2], Mariana dos Santos Dutra Okada[1], Otávia Reis e Silva[3], Joaquim Esquerdo Ferreira[4] and Marco Roberto Bourg de Mello[1*]

1 Universidade Federal Rural do Rio de Janeiro (UFRRJ), Seropedica, RJ, Brasil

2 Universidade de Barra Mansa (UBM), Barra Mansa, RJ, Brasil

3 Univassouras, Vassouras, RJ, Brasil

4 Centro Universitário de Valença (UNIFAA), Valença, RJ, Brasil

*Address all correspondence to: mmrural@gmail.com

References

[1] Fernandez-Novo A, Santos-Lopez S, Pesantez-Pacheco JL, Pérez-Villalobos N, Heras-Molina A, Gonzalez-Martin JV, et al. Effects on synchronization and reproductive efficiency of delaying the removal of the intravaginal progesterone device by 24 h in the 5d co-synch protocol in heifers. Animals. 2021;**11**(3):849. DOI: 10.3390/ani11030849

[2] Cardoso Consentini CE, Wiltbank MC, Sartori R. Factors that optimize reproductive efficiency in dairy herds with an emphasis on timed artificial insemination programs. Animals. 2021;**11**(2):301. DOI: 10.3390/ani11020301

[3] Pugliesi G, Oliveria M, Scolari S, Lopes E, Pinaffi F, Miagawa B, et al. Corpus luteum development and function after supplementation of long-acting progesterone during the early luteal phase in beef cattle. Reproduction in Domestic Animals. 2014;**49**(1):85-91. DOI: 10.1111/rda.12231

[4] Lonergan P, Forde N, Spencer T. Role of progesterone in embryo development in cattle. Reproduction, Fertility, and Development. 2016;**28**(2):66. DOI: 10.1071/rd15326

[5] Amado JA, Floréz J. Hormonas sexuales: estrógenos, gestágenos, andrógenos y anticonceptivos hormonales. 4a ed. Barcelona: Masson; 2003. 887 p

[6] Hafez B, Hafez ES, editores. Reproduction in Farm Animals. Baltimore, Maryland, USA: Lippincott Williams & Wilkins; 2000. DOI: 10.1002/9781119265306

[7] Wiltbank MC, Souza AH, Carvalho PD, Cunha AP, Giordano JO, Fricke PM, et al. Physiological and practical effects of progesterone on reproduction in dairy cattle. Animal. 2014;**8**:70-81. DOI: 10.1017/s1751731114000585

[8] Rigoglio NN, Fátima LA, Hanassaka JY, Pinto GL, Machado AS, Gimenes LU, et al. Equine chorionic gonadotropin alters luteal cell morphologic features related to progesterone synthesis. Theriogenology. 2013;**79**(4):673-679. DOI: 10.1016/j.theriogenology.2012.11.023

[9] Binelli M, Pugliesi G, Batista EO, Martins T, Lopes E, Sponchiado M, et al. Uterine receptivity and fertility programming in beef cows. Revista Brasileira de Reprodução Animal. 2017;**41**(1):121-129

[10] Clemente M, de La Fuente J, Fair T, Al Naib A, Gutierrez-Adan A, Roche JF, et al. Progesterone and conceptus elongation in cattle: a direct effect on the embryo or an indirect effect via the endometrium? Reproduction. 2009;**138**(3):507-517. DOI: 10.1530/rep-09-0152

[11] Meneghetti M, Filho OG, Peres RF, Lamb GC, Vasconcelos JL. Fixed-time artificial insemination with estradiol and progesterone for Bos indicus cows I: Basis for development of protocols. Theriogenology. 2009;**72**(2):179-189. DOI: 10.1016/j.theriogenology.2009.02.010

[12] Yan L, Robinson R, Shi Z, Mann G. Efficacy of progesterone supplementation during early pregnancy in cows: A meta-analysis. Theriogenology. 2016;**85**(8):1390-1398. DOI: 10.1016/j.theriogenology.2015.12.027

[13] de Graaff W, Grimard B. Progesterone-releasing devices for cattle estrus induction and synchronization: Device optimization to anticipate shorter treatment durations and new device developments. Theriogenology. 2018;**112**:34-43. DOI: 10.1016/j.theriogenology.2017.09.025

[14] Spencer T, Bazer F. Uterine and placental factors regulating conceptus growth in domestic animals. Journal of Animal Science. 2004;**82**:E4e13. DOI: 10.2527/2004.8213_supplE4x

[15] Adeyemo O, Heath E. Plasma progesterone concentration in Bos taurus and Bos indicus heifers. Theriogenology. 1980;**14**(6):411-420. DOI: 10.1016/0093-691x(80)90052-7

[16] Badinga L, Thatcher WW, Wilcox CJ, Morris G, Entwistle K, Wolfenson D. Effect of season on follicular dynamics and plasma concentrations of estradiol-17β, progesterone and luteinizing hormone in lactating Holstein cows. Theriogenology. 1994;**42**(8):1263-1274. DOI: 10.1016/0093-691x(94)90246-f

[17] Bazer FW. Uterine receptivity to implantation of blastocysts in mammals. Frontiers in Bioscience. 2011;**S3**(2):745-767. DOI: 10.2741/s184

[18] Kenyon AG, Mendonça LGD, Lopes G, Lima JR, Santos JEP, Chebel RC. Minimal progesterone concentration is required for embryo survival after embryo transfer in lactating Holstein cows. Animal Reproduction Science. 2013;**136**(4):223-230. DOI: 10.1016/j.anireprosci.2012.10.014

[19] Lonergan P. Influence of progesterone on oocyte quality and embryo development in cows. Theriogenology. 2011;**76**(9):1594-1601. DOI: 10.1016/j.theriogenology.2011.06.012

[20] Nascimento AB, Bender RW, Souza AH, Ayres H, Araujo RR, Guenther JN, et al. Effect of treatment with human chorionic gonadotropin on day 5 after timed artificial insemination on fertility of lactating dairy cows. Journal of Dairy Science. 2013;**96**(5):2873-2882. DOI: 10.3168/jds.2012-5895

[21] Pugliesi G, Santos FB, Lopes E, Nogueira É, Maio JRG, Binelli M. Fertility response in suckled beef cows supplemented with long-acting progesterone after timed artificial insemination. Reproduction, Fertility and Development. 2015;**27**(1):98. DOI: 10.1071/RDv27n1Ab11

[22] Junior WMC, Cooke RF, Pereira MHC, Vasconcelos JLM. Effects of melengestrol acetate supplementation after fixed-timed artificial insemination on pregnancy rates of Bos indicus beef cows. Livestock Science. 2017;**206**:71-75. DOI: 10.1016/j.livsci.2017.10.012

[23] Ball PJH, Peters AR. Reproduction in Cattle. Oxford, UK; Ames, Iowa: Blackwell Pub; 2014

[24] Perry GA. Factors affecting puberty in replacement beef heifers. Theriogenology. 2016;**86**(1):373-378. DOI: 10.1016/j.theriogenology.2016.04.051

[25] Lima RS, Martins T, Lemes KM, Binelli M, Madureira EH. Effect of a puberty induction protocol based on injectable long acting progesterone on pregnancy success of beef heifers serviced by TAI. Theriogenology. 2020;**154**:128-134. DOI: 10.1016/j.theriogenology.2020.05.036

[26] Sá Filho MF, Nasser LFT, Penteado L, Prestes R, Marques MO, Freitas BG, et al. Impact of progesterone and estradiol treatment before the onset

of the breeding period on reproductive performance of Bos indicus beef heifers. Animal Reproduction Science. 2015;**1**(160):30-39. DOI: 10.1016/j.anireprosci.2015.06.024

[27] Patterson DJ, Thomas JM, Martin NT, Nash JM, Smith MF. Control of estrus and ovulation in beef heifers. Veterinary Clinics of North America: Food Animal Practice. 2013;**29**(3):591-617. DOI: 10.1016/j.cvfa.2013.07.009

[28] de Araújo AC, Nonato MS, ARA B, DCRX M, DVF M, JML S. Induction of ovulation in heifers with memorandum of cyclicality. Brazilian Journal of Development. 2019;**5**(11):24286-24290. DOI: 10.34117/bjdv5n11-115

[29] Ireland JJ, Roche JF. Effect of progesterone on basal LH and episodic LH and FSH secretion in heifers. Reproduction. 1982;**64**(2):295-302. DOI: 10.1530/jrf.0.0640295

[30] Blache D, Fabre-Nys C, Venier G. Ventromedial hypothalamus as a target for oestradiol action on proceptivity, receptivity and luteinizing hormone surge of the ewe. Brains. Research. 1991;**546**(2):241-249. DOI: 10.1016/0006-8993(91)91488-M

[31] Claro Júnior I, Filho OGS, Peres RFG, Aono FHS, Day ML, Vasconcelos JLM. Reproductive performance of prepubertal Bos indicus heifers after progesterone-based treatments. Theriogenology. 2010;**74**(6):903-911. DOI: 10.1016/j.theriogenology.2010.04.015

[32] Taraborrelli S. Physiology, production and action of progesterone. Acta Obstetricia et Gynecologica Scandinavica. 2015;**S161**:8-16. DOI: 10.1111/aogs.12771

[33] Anderson LH, Mcdowell CM, Day ML. Progestin-induced puberty and secretion of luteinizing hormone in heifers. Biology of Reproduction. 1996;**54**:1025e31. DOI: 10.1095/biolreprod54.5.1025

[34] Vrisman DP, Bastos NM, Rossi GF, Rodrigues NN, Borges LPB, Taira AR, et al. Corpus luteum dynamics after ovulation induction with or without previous exposure to progesterone in prepubertal Nellore heifers. Theriogenology. 2018;**106**:60-68. DOI: 10.1016/j.theriogenology.2017.10.018

[35] Rodrigues P, Peres G, Lemes AP, Martins T, Pereira C, Carvalho ER, et al. Effect of interval from induction of puberty to initiation of a timed AI protocol on pregnancy rate in Nellore heifers. Theriogenology. 2014;**82**(5):760-766. DOI: 10.1016/j.theriogenology.2014.06.008

[36] Mann G, Lamming G. Relationship between maternal endocrine environment, early embryo development and inhibition of the luteolytic mechanism in cows. Reproduction. 2001;**121**(1):175-180

[37] Forde N, Beltman ME, Duffy GB, Duffy P, Mehta JP, O'Gaora P, et al. Changes in the endometrial transcriptome during the bovine estrous cycle: effect of low circulating progesterone and consequences for conceptus elongation. Biology of Reproduction. 2010;**84**(2):266-278. DOI: 10.1095/biolreprod.110.085910

[38] Pugliesi G, Santos FB, Lopes E, Nogueira MJRG, Binelli M. Improved fertility in suckled beef cows ovulating large follicles or supplemented with long-acting progesterone after timed-AI. Theriogenology. 2016;**85**:1239-1248. DOI: 10.1016/j.theriogenology.2015.12.006

[39] Garcia-Ispierto I, López-Gatius F. Progesterone supplementation in the early

luteal phase after artificial insemination improves pregnancy rates in high-producing dairy cows. Theriogenology. 2017;**90**:20-24. DOI: 10.1016/j.theriogenology.2016.11.006

[40] Ababneh MM, Alnimer MA, Husein MQ. Effect of post insemination progesterone supplement on pregnancy rates of repeat breeder friesian cows. Asian-Australasian Journal of Animal Sciences. 2007;**20**(11):1670-1676. DOI: 10.5713/ajas.2007.1670

[41] Mehni SB, Shabankareh HK, Kazemi-Bonchenari M, Eghbali M. The comparison of treating holstein dairy cows with progesterone, CIDR and GnRH after insemination on serum progesterone and pregnancy rates. Reproduction in Domestic Animals. 2012;**47**:131-134. DOI: 10.1111/j.1439-0531.2011.01811.x

[42] Parr MH, Crowe MA, Lonergan P, Evans A, Rizos D, Diskin MG. Effect of exogenous progesterone supplementation in the early luteal phase post-insemination on pregnancy per artificial insemination in Holstein–Friesian cows. Animal Reproduction Science. 2014;**150**(1-2):7-14. DOI: 10.1016/j.anireprosci.2014.08.008

[43] Parr MH, Scully S, Lonergan P, Evans ACO, Crowe MA, Diskin MG. Establishment of critical timing of progesterone supplementation on corpus luteum and embryo development in beef heifers. Animal Reproduction Science. 2017;**180**:1-9. DOI: 10.1016/j.anireprosci.2017.02.005

[44] Silva KM, Leão MC, Rodrigues TC, Marques N, Antônio M. Administration of GnRH on the day of fixed-time artificial insemination (FTAI) and melengestrol acetate (MGA) administration after FTAI in non-suckling Nelore cattle. Semina Ciências Agrárias. 2015;**36**(5):3149-3149. DOI: 10.5433/1679-0359.2015v36n5p3149

[45] Johnson KR, Ross RH, Fourt DL. Effect of progesterone administration on reproductive efficiency. Journal of Animal Science. 1958;**17**(2):386-390. DOI: 10.2527/jas1958.172386x

[46] Couto SRB, Guerson YB, Ferreira JE, Silva OR, Silenciato LN, Barbero RP, et al. Impact of supplementation with long-acting progesterone on gestational loss in Nelore females submitted to TAI. Theriogenology. 2019;**125**:168-172. DOI: 10.1016/j.theriogenology.2018.10.032

[47] Couto SRB, Guerson YB, Caparelli NMPM, Jacob AJPN, JCF, Barbero RP, Mello MRB. Mitigation of low pregnancy rate in excitable Nellore cows by administration of GnRH or P4. Theriogenology. 2022;**192**:14-21. DOI: 10.1016/j.theriogenology.2022.08.003

[48] Mann G, Lamming G. The influence of progesterone during early pregnancy in cattle. Reproduction in Domestic Animals. 1999;**34**(3-4):269-274. DOI: 10.1111/j.1439-0531.1999.tb01250.x

[49] O'Hara L, Forde N, Carter F, Rizos D, Maillo V, Ealy AD, et al. Paradoxical effect of supplementary progesterone between day 3 and day 7 on corpus luteum function and conceptus development in cattle. Reproduction, Fertility and Development. 2014;**26**(2):328-328. DOI: 10.1071/RD12370

[50] Martins T, Pugliesi G, Sponchiado M, Cardoso BO, Gomes NS, Mello BP, et al. Supplementation with long-acting progesterone in early diestrus in beef cattle: I. effect of artificial insemination on onset of luteolysis. Domestic Animal Endocrinology. 2019;**67**:63-70. Available

from: https://www.sciencedirect.com/science/article/pii/S0739724018300882

[51] Binelli M, Sartori R, Vasconcelos JLM, Monteiro PLJ, Pereira MHC, Ramos RS. Evolution in fixed-time: from synchronization of ovulation to improved fertility. Bioscientifica Proceedings. 2019;**8**:RDRRDR34. DOI: 10.1530/biosciprocs.8.034

[52] Bech-Sàbat G, López-Gatius F, García-Ispierto I, Santolaria JP, Serrano B, Nogareda C, et al. Pregnancy patterns during the early fetal period in high producing dairy cows treated with GnRH or progesterone. Theriogenology. 2009;**71**(6):920-929. DOI: 10.1016/j.theriogenology.2008.10.013

[53] Beltran MP, Vasconcelos JLM. Conception rate in Holstein cows treated with GnRH or hCG on the fifth day post artificial insemination during summer. Arquivo Brasileiro de Medicina Veterinária e Zootecnia. 2008;**60**(3):580-586. DOI: 10.1590/S0102-09352008000300009

[54] Thatcher WW, Guzeloglu A, Meikle A, Kamimura S, Bilby T, Kowalski AA, et al. Regulation of embryo survival in cattle. Reproduction Supplement. 2003;**61**:253-266

[55] Besbaci M, Abdelli A, Minviel JJ, Belabdi I, Kaidi R, Raboisson D. Association of pregnancy per artificial insemination with gonadotropin-releasing hormone and human chorionic gonadotropin administered during the luteal phase after artificial insemination in dairy cows: A meta-analysis. Journal of Dairy Science. 2020;**103**:2006-2018. DOI: 10.3168/jds.2019-16439

[56] Dahlen CR, Bird SL, Martel CA, Olson K, Stevenson JS, Lamb GC. Administration of human chorionic gonadotropin 7 days after fixed-time artificial insemination of suckled beef cows1. Journal of Animal Science. 2010;**88**(7):2337-2345. DOI: 10.2527/jas.2009-2596

[57] Stevenson JS, Portaluppi MA, Tenhouse DE, Lloyd A, Eborn DR, Kacuba S, et al. Interventions after artificial insemination: conception rates, pregnancy survival, and ovarian responses to gonadotropin-releasing hormone, human chorionic gonadotropin, and progesterone. Journal of Dairy Science. 2007;**90**(1):331-340. DOI: 10.3168/jds.S0022-0302(07)72634-6

[58] Araújo RR, Ginther OJ, Ferreira JC, Palhão MM, Beg MA, Wiltbank MC. Role of follicular estradiol-17 beta in timing of luteolysis in heifers1. Biology of Reproduction. 2009;**81**(2):426-437. DOI: 10.1095/biolreprod.108.073825

[59] Lòpez-Gatius F, Santolaria P, Martino A, Delétang F, Rensis F. The effects of GnRH treatment at the time of AI and 12 days later on reproductive performance of high producing dairy cows during the warm season in northeastern Spain. Theriogenology. 2006;**65**(4):820-830. DOI: 10.1016/j.theriogenology.2005.07.002

[60] Howard JM, Manzo R, Dalton JC, Frago F, Ahmadzadeh A. Conception rates and serum progesterone concentration in dairy cattle administered gonadotropin releasing hormone 5 days after artificial insemination. Animal Reproduction Science. 2006;**95**:224-233. DOI: 10.1016/j.anireprosci.2005.10.010

[61] Ataman MB, Erdem H, Bülbül B, Ümütlü S, Çolak M. The effect of buserelin injection 12 days after insemination on selected reproductive characteristics in cows. Acta Veterinaria.

2011;**80**:171-177. DOI: 10.2754/avb201180020171

[62] Pinto TLC, Nogueira MBR, Sales JN, Carvalho RR, Cushman RA, Souza JC. Fatores afetando as taxas de gestação após a transferência de embriões derivados de aspiração folicular em receptoras Holstein lactantes sob condições tropicais. Cienc. e Agrotecnologia. 2015;**39**:498-505. DOI: 10.1590/S1413-70542015000500008

[63] Stojanov B, Atanasov B, Grizelj J, Vince S, Nikolovski M, Kjosevski M, et al. Induction and formation of accessory corpus luteum after artificial insemination (AI) might increase pregnancy rate per AI in heat stressed dairy cows. Macedonian Veterinary Review. 2020;**43**:37-43. DOI: 10.2478/macvetrev-2020-0012

[64] Akhtar MS, Saleem M, Ahmad E, Ahmad T, Lashari MH, Ayaz MM, et al. Effect of lecirelin acetate, hcg or progesterone administration on day 7 post-insemination on conception rate and progesterone concentration in cross-bred cattle. Iraqi Journal of Veterinary Sciences. 2018;**32**:149-153. DOI: 10.33899/ijvs.2019.153842

[65] Baez GM, Trevisol E, Barletta RV, Cardoso BO, Ricci A, Guenther JN, et al. Proposal of a new model for CL regression or maintenance during pregnancy on the basis of timing of regression of contralateral, accessory CL in pregnant cows. Theriogenology. 2017;**89**:214-225. DOI: 10.1016/j.theriogenology.2016.09.055

[66] Monteiro PLJ, Sartori R, Canavessi AMO, Melo LF, Motta JCL, Consentini CEC, et al. Accessory corpus lutem regression during pregnancy I: timing, physiology, and P4 profiles. Reproduction. 2021;**162**:473-482. DOI: 10.1530/REP-21-0167

[67] Monteiro PLJ, Gamarra CA, Genari RS, Prata AB, Barletta RV, Duran PG, et al. Accessory corpus lutem regression during pregnancy II: reproductive outcomes. Reproduction. 2021;**162**:483-495. DOI: 10.1530/REP-21-0168